THE ART OF HOME APOTHECARY

Natural Remedies and Step-by-Step Guides for Healing, Daily Wellness, and Family Health

ScriptoraLab

COPYRIGHT

DISCLAIMER

This book is intended solely for educational and informational purposes. The information contained herein is based on research, personal experiences, and traditional knowledge regarding the use of medicinal herbs and should not be considered a substitute for professional medical advice, diagnosis, or treatment.

Reader Responsibility:
The author is not a certified medical doctor or healthcare professional and cannot provide personalized medical advice. Before using any natural remedy or medicinal herb described in this book, it is essential to consult your doctor or a qualified healthcare provider, especially if:

- *You are pregnant or breastfeeding.*
- *You have pre-existing medical conditions.*
- *You are taking prescription or over-the-counter medications.*
- *You have known allergies to plants or botanical ingredients.*

Use of Natural Remedies:
The use of medicinal herbs can carry risks, particularly if used in inappropriate dosages or in combination with medications. Not all herbs are safe for everyone. Natural remedies must be used cautiously, following the recommended dosages and closely monitoring individual reactions. Discontinue the use of any remedy immediately in the event of adverse effects and consult a medical professional.

No Guarantee of Effectiveness:
The information in this book is provided "as is," and the author makes no guarantees regarding the specific results or effectiveness of any remedy described. Each individual is unique and may respond differently to herbs and natural treatments.

Limitation of Liability:
The author assumes no responsibility for direct, indirect, incidental, or consequential damages resulting from the use, application, or interpretation of the information contained in this book. The reader is solely responsible for decisions related to their health and well-being.

Informed Consent:
By using the information in this book, the reader agrees to take full responsibility for the use of the remedies and techniques described, understanding the potential risks and benefits.

Consultation with Experts:
This book cannot replace the advice of a doctor, pharmacist, or qualified herbalist. For urgent or critical medical situations, consult a healthcare professional immediately.

Ongoing Research:
Knowledge in the fields of herbalism and medicine is constantly evolving. Readers are encouraged to stay informed about new scientific discoveries and updates regarding herbs and natural remedies.

CONCLUSION

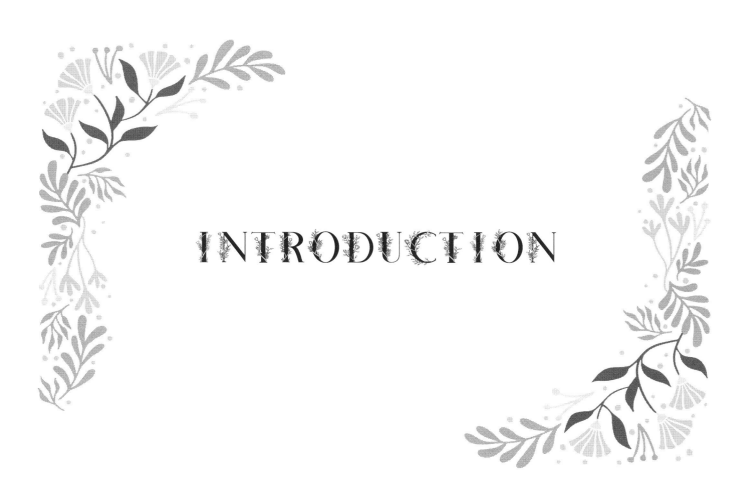

INTRODUCTION

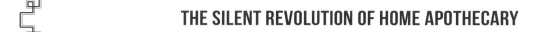
THE HISTORY OF THE HOME APOTHECARY: A JOURNEY FROM ANCIENT TRADITIONS TO MODERN PRACTICES

Home apothecary is more than just a practice: it is a deep connection between man and nature, a way to rediscover ancient traditions and adapt them to modern needs. This quiet revolution was not born today; it has its roots in distant eras, when knowledge of plants and natural remedies was an integral part of daily life.

Millennia ago, primitive communities learned to observe nature, discovering that certain plants could relieve pain, heal wounds and even save lives. In the absence of modern doctors or pharmacies, it was the women and village elders who guarded and passed on this valuable knowledge. The ancient Egyptians, for example, used aloe vera to treat burns, while the Chinese compiled detailed texts such as the "Shennong Bencao Jing," a compendium of medicinal herbs written over 2,000 years ago.

In the Western world, the Greeks and Romans were among the first to systematize herbal medicine. Hippocrates, considered the father of medicine, taught that nature itself is the best cure for disease. Galen, a Roman physician, perfected the preparation of ointments and decoctions that today we would consider the ancestors of modern ointments. During the Middle Ages, however, much of this knowledge remained in the hands of monks and apothecaries. Monasteries became true centers of botanical research, where herbs were cultivated and recipes were transcribed in so-called "herbaria."

In the Renaissance, home apothecary got a new impetus. With the spread of printing, books such as John Gerard's "Herbal" allowed herbal knowledge to reach even ordinary households. People began to make herbal teas, tinctures and ointments at home, turning the kitchen into a laboratory. Women, in particular, played a central role: they were the ones who gathered herbs, prepared remedies, and treated family members.

However, with the arrival of modern medicine in the 19th century, the importance of the home apothecary began to decline. New scientific discoveries led to the emergence of faster and more effective synthetic drugs, and the ancient practice of natural cures was often relegated to a secondary role, seen as antiquated or unreliable. But as conventional medicine spread, many rural communities and cultural groups continued to pass on the secrets of herbs, keeping the tradition alive.

In recent decades, a change has become evident: the home apothecary is experiencing a renaissance. Growing awareness of the side effects of industrial drugs, interest in a sustainable lifestyle, and the desire to reduce dependence on chemicals have prompted many people to rediscover the power of plants. This revolution, while quiet, is deeply rooted in the human need to connect with nature and care for their bodies in a kind and respectful way.

Today, creating a home apothecary means not only recovering ancient wisdom but also adapting it to the needs of modern life. You can combine current science with traditional knowledge, using simple tools such as mortar and pestle along with modern technologies such as desiccators. You do not need to be an expert botanist to get started: with a little curiosity and dedication, anyone can learn how to prepare effective and safe remedies for themselves and their loved ones.

This practice is not only therapeutic: it is also a way to cultivate gratitude to nature. Every plant grown in the garden, every herbal tea prepared with care, represents a step toward a more balanced and harmonious life. The home apothecary is not just a collection of herbs and recipes; it is a bridge between the past and the present, a conscious choice for a healthier and more sustainable future.

In the next chapter, we explore the essential tools for building your own home apothecary, discovering how to organize your space and begin cultivating this ancient art.

THE IMPORTANCE OF RETURNING TO NATURE: BENEFITS FOR HEALTH, ENVIRONMENT AND MENTAL WELLBEING

In the modern era, we often find ourselves immersed in a hectic lifestyle that is increasingly distant from nature. This detachment is not without consequences: chronic stress, environmental pollution, and an increase in diseases related to unhealthy lifestyles are just some of the problems that characterize our time. Returning to nature, rediscovering practices such as home apothecary, is a concrete and meaningful response to these challenges.

From a health perspective, the use of natural remedies makes it possible to reduce exposure to synthetic drugs and their potential side effects. Medicinal plants, properly used, offer a gentle but effective alternative for treating common ailments such as insomnia, headaches or digestive problems. In addition, preparing home remedies allows us to know and choose carefully what we use, giving us back control over our health.

Environmentally, growing our own medicinal herbs or buying natural ingredients from local producers reduces the ecological impact associated with the industrial production of medicines and cosmetics. Making an ointment or tincture at home also means avoiding unnecessary packaging and reducing waste, contributing to a more sustainable lifestyle. Each plant grown in our garden or balcony becomes a small step toward a more balanced relationship with the planet.

Finally, the benefits to mental well-being are profound and immediate. The simple act of working with plants-sowing, harvesting, drying-fosters an authentic connection with nature, reducing stress and improving mood. The practice of home apothecary is inherently meditative: it requires attention, calm and care, turning each preparation into a moment of presence and gratitude.

In an increasingly complex world, returning to nature is an invitation to slow down, take care of ourselves and live more mindfully. It is a healing path not only for the body, but also for the mind and soul.

HOW THIS BOOK CAN GUIDE YOU STEP-BY-STEP IN CREATING YOUR HEALING CORNER

Creating a home apothecary is a fascinating journey, but it can seem complex when you first start. What herbs to choose? What tools are needed? How to store and use the remedies safely? This book is designed to answer all these questions, offering you a practical and accessible guide to turning a corner of your home into a space dedicated to natural health. Each chapter will take you through a step-by-step process, starting with the basics and ending with more advanced preparations. We'll start with the basics: what tools are essential, how to organize your space, and what medicinal plants to grow or buy to get started. You don't need to have a garden or extensive knowledge: this book is designed to fit any lifestyle, whether you live in the country, the city or an apartment.

Once the basics are set, we will delve into the heart of home apothecary: learning how to prepare tinctures, infused oils, ointments, herbal teas, and other remedies using simple but effective techniques. Each step is explained in detail and accompanied by proven recipes that you can customize to suit your needs and preferences.

This book not only teaches you how to create remedies, but also helps you understand the properties of plants, their benefits, and the precautions necessary for safe use. In addition, you'll find more than 250 herbal remedies to address common ailments, so you'll always have a natural solution at your fingertips.

More than a practical guide, this book is an invitation to build a deep and conscious relationship with nature. It will encourage you to explore, experiment and find joy in the process of creation, turning your healing corner into a source of well-being not only for you, but also for those around you.

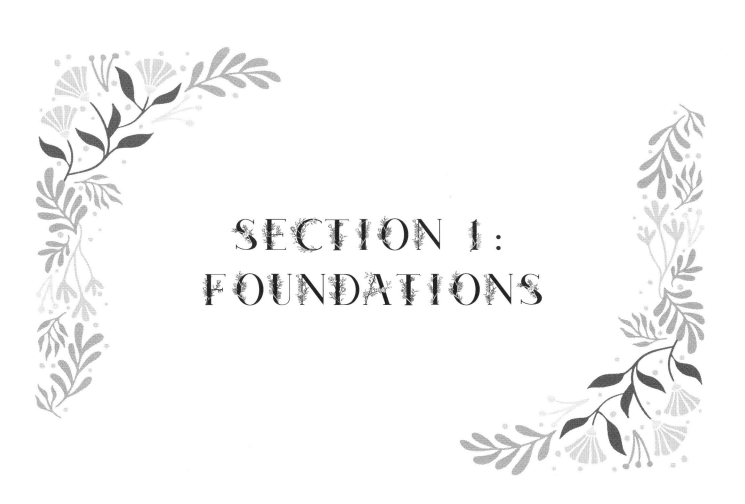

SECTION 1: FOUNDATIONS

CHAPTER 1:
THE ESSENTIAL TOOLS OF THE HOME APOTHECARY

The home apothecary is a natural wellness laboratory, and like any laboratory, it requires essential tools to be effective and organized. Building your basic kit is not complicated, and many of the necessary items are already present in homes. With these tools, preparing remedies such as tinctures, infused oils, herbal teas, and ointments will be a pleasure.

Basic Equipment

- **Mortar and pestle**: Essential for grinding fresh or dried herbs and breaking down hard seeds. Choose a ceramic or granite mortar for durability and convenience.
- **Glass jars**: Used to store dried herbs, tinctures and infused oils. Prefer airtight jars with dark glass to protect contents from light.
- **Filters**: Muslins, steel strainers and paper filters are essential for separating liquids from the solid parts of herbs. A reusable muslin is an environmentally friendly choice.
- **Drippers and droppers**: Perfect for dispensing tinctures or essential oils precisely. Prefer droppers with good quality rubber caps for long-term use.
- **Precision scales**: Optional but very useful, especially for dosing small amounts of herbs or ingredients.

These tools not only make the preparation process more efficient, but also ensure that your remedies are safe and well stored. Start with what you already have and expand your kit gradually.

Checklist for your first kit

- ☐ Mortar and pestle
- ☐ Glass jars
- ☐ Strainers or gauze
- ☐ Steel pot
- ☐ Sticky labels
- ☐ Digital scale

With this kit and a well-organized space, you are ready to begin your journey into home apothecary. In the next chapter we will explore the most useful medicinal herbs to get you started, learning how to choose and recognize the right ones for your needs.

Did you know?

The mortar and pestle are among humanity's oldest tools, used since prehistoric times to grind herbs, grains and spices. Their shape has not changed much over the centuries!

SPACE ORGANIZATION: CREATING A SAFE AND PRACTICAL ENVIRONMENT FOR WORKING

A well-organized home pharmacy not only makes it easier to prepare remedies, but also ensures safety and practicality. Your space does not have to be large; it can be a shelf, a cabinet, or a part of the kitchen, as long as it is well structured.

1. The Ideal Location
Choose a cool, dry place away from direct sunlight to store herbs and tools. Light and moisture can impair the effectiveness of herbs and alter preparations. If possible, dedicate a dedicated shelf or cabinet, preferably near a clean, stable work surface.

2. Organization of Tools
- Jars and containers: Label each jar with the name of the plant, date of harvest or preparation, and expiration date. Use water-resistant labels.
- Tools: Store your mortar, pestles and strainers in a separate drawer or box to keep them clean and protected from dust.
- Small equipment: Use divider boxes for droppers, strainers and other small tools.

3. Space for Preparations

Dedicate a clean and neat work surface for remedy preparation. Make sure it is easy to clean and away from food or incompatible substances.

4. Safety
- Keep out of reach of children: Store tinctures and essential oils in a high or enclosed place.
- Emergency supplies: Keep a clean cloth and alcohol on hand to clean up any spills.

5. Ideas for small spaces
- Use a cart with wheels to create a mobile pharmacy. You can move it easily and make the most of the available space.
- Install vertical shelves to store jars and tools without taking up valuable floor space.

Did you know?

In the Middle Ages, herbalists organized their remedies in shelves divided by "seasons" or "elements" (earth, water, air, fire). Today we can draw inspiration from this logic to organize herbs by use: digestive, relaxing, skin, etc.

Checklist for your perfect space:

☐ Shelf or cabinet away from direct light

☐ Labeled and tightly closed containers

☐ Clean surface dedicated to preparations

☐ Silica gel bags or absorbent clay to reduce moisture

With smart and functional organization, your space will become a corner of peace and creativity, where every remedy will be prepared with care and precision.

ADVANCED ACCESSORIES: DESICCATORS, ESSENTIAL OIL DISTILLERS, PRECISION SCALES

When you are ready to take your home pharmacy to the next level, some advanced accessories can help you achieve more professional results. Although not essential to get started, these tools give you greater precision, efficiency, and the ability to experiment with more complex preparations.

1. Dryers

A dryer is a valuable tool for preserving herbs quickly and effectively, especially in humid environments where natural drying can be more difficult.

- Advantages:
    - o Reduces drying time compared to traditional methods.
    - o Keeps active properties of herbs intact through controlled temperatures.

- What to look for in a dryer:
    - o A model with adjustable temperature, preferably with a range between 30-50°C.
    - o Removable trays for drying different amounts of herbs.

- Alternatives:
    - o If you don't have a dryer, a low-temperature oven with the door slightly open may be an option, although less efficient.

2. Essential Oil Distillers

If you love essential oils and want to make them at home, a distiller is an indispensable tool. This accessory allows you to extract pure oils from herbs such as lavender, mint, and rosemary.

- How it works:
    - o The distiller uses steam to separate essential oils from plants.
    - o It requires some practice to get the right balance between amounts of herbs and water.

- Benefits:
    - o Fresh, high-quality essential oils.
    - o Ability to create unique and customized blends.

- Tip for beginners:
    - o Start with small distillers to experiment without excessive investment.

3. Precision Scales

A precision scale is essential for accurately dosing quantities of herbs, oils and solvents. This is especially important for tinctures, ointments, and creams where proportions affect the safety and efficacy of the remedy.

- What to look for in a scale:
    - o Accuracy down to 0.1 gram.
    - o Digital models that are easy to read and use.
    - o Tare function for weighing with containers.

- Practical Tip:
    - o Use a separate scale to weigh dry herbs and liquid oils to maintain cleanliness and accuracy.

When to invest in advanced accessories:

- If you have started preparing remedies regularly and want to improve quality and efficiency.
- When you want to explore advanced preparations, such as distillation or complex infused oils.

You don't need everything right away! Start with the basic tools and consider advanced accessories only when you feel you really need them. Enthusiasm is important, but a step-by-step approach will help you avoid unnecessary expense.

By introducing these advanced accessories, you can take your home pharmacy to a professional level, expanding the creative possibilities and preparations available.

CHAPTER 2:
MEDICINAL PLANTS: BASIC KNOWLEDGE

Discovering the world of medicinal plants is like opening a door to a realm of millennia-old traditions and endless possibilities. Each plant tells a story, and its use for health and wellness represents a deep connection between humans and nature. For a beginner, getting started may seem like a daunting task, given the huge number of plants available and their variety of uses. However, some herbs stand out for their versatility, safety and ease of use, making them ideal for building the foundation of your home pharmacy.

THE IMPORTANCE OF BASIC MEDICINAL PLANTS

Medicinal plants are not only useful for dealing with minor ailments, but can also be integrated into a daily routine to promote optimal health. For those starting out, it is essential to become familiar with plants that are effective and relatively simple to use. These herbs provide a good starting point, not only because of their healing effects but also because they offer a practical introduction to harvesting, drying, and preparation techniques.

Herb selection should be based on a few key considerations: local availability, ease of cultivation and storage, and their ability to address a variety of common ailments. Below is an in-depth guide to some of the most useful herbs for beginners.

KNOWING HERBS: A REFERENCE CHART

To make it easier to understand and use medicinal plants, I have created a table listing some of the most beginner-friendly herbs. Each herb is described with its common name, botanical name, main properties, and methods of use.

Common Name	Botanical name	Main Properties	Parts Used	Common Uses
Marigold	Calendula officinalis	Anti-inflammatory, healing	Flowers	Wounds, skin irritations, ointments
Mint	Mentha piperita	Digestive, refreshing	Leaves	Herbal teas for nausea, oil for headaches
Chamomile	Matricaria chamomilla	Calming, antispasmodic	Flowers	Infusions for anxiety, sleep, intestinal cramps
Lavender	Lavandula angustifolia	Relaxing, antiseptic	Flowers	Oils for stress, herbal teas for insomnia
Thyme	Thymus vulgaris	Antibacterial, expectorant	Leaves and flowers	Herbal teas for coughs, inhalations for colds
Sage	Salvia officinalis	Astringent, antiseptic	Leaves	Gargles for sore throats, toning herbal teas

Common Name	Botanical name	Main Properties	Parts Used	Common Uses
Melissa	Melissa officinalis	Sedative, antiviral	Leaves	Herbal teas for anxiety, insomnia, chapped lips
Ginger	Zingiber officinale	Anti-inflammatory, digestive	Rhizome	Infusions for nausea, muscle pain
Echinacea	Echinacea purpurea	Immunostimulant	Roots, flowers	Herbal teas for colds, defense tinctures
Rosemary	Rosmarinus officinalis	Stimulant, antioxidant	Leaves	Massage oils, energizing herbal teas
Yarrow	Achillea millefolium	Anti-inflammatory, astringent	Flowers and leaves	Herbal teas for menstrual pain, wounds
St. John's wort	Hypericum perforatum	Antidepressant, antiseptic	Flowers	Oils for irritated skin, herbal teas for mood
Fennel	Foeniculum vulgare	Digestive, antispasmodic	Seeds	Infusions for swelling, herbal teas for colic
Aloe Vera	Aloe barbadensis	Soothing, hydrating	Gel from the leaves	Gel for burns, skin irritations
Dandelion	Taraxacum officinale	Purifying, diuretic	Roots, leaves, flowers	Herbal teas for liver, digestion

DETAILED DESCRIPTION OF SELECTED HERBS

Calendula (Calendula officinalis)

Calendula is often considered the queen of skin care plants. Its orange and golden flowers contain powerful anti-inflammatory compounds that promote healing of wounds, cuts and skin irritations. It is an easy plant to grow and versatile to use. It can be made into ointments, infused oils or simply used in decoctions for rinses.

Mint (Mentha piperita)

Mint is one of the most familiar and accessible herbs. It is excellent for digestive disorders such as nausea, bloating and poor digestion. The infusion of mint leaves is a quick and effective remedy to calm the stomach. In addition, mint essential oil is useful for relieving headaches and muscle tension.

Chamomile (Matricaria chamomilla)

A classic calming remedy, chamomile is known for its antispasmodic and soothing properties. Chamomile infusions are ideal for promoting sleep, reducing stress and relieving abdominal cramps. It is an herb that lends itself to many uses, including eye compresses for tired eyes.

Lavender (Lavandula angustifolia)

Lavender is the symbol of serenity. Its purple flowers, besides being visually appealing, produce an essential oil rich in relaxing and antiseptic benefits. It can be used in herbal teas, aromatic baths and diffusers to promote a sense of calm and well-being.

Thyme (Thymus vulgaris)

Thyme is a powerful plant for fighting respiratory infections due to its antibacterial and expectorant properties. An infusion of thyme is an excellent remedy for coughs and sore throats, while thyme inhalations help clear the respiratory tract. It is a hardy plant that is easy to grow, and its benefits are as ancient as they are effective.

Sage (Salvia officinalis)

Known for its Latin name, meaning "to save," sage is a highly versatile herb. It is especially useful as an antiseptic for oral problems, such as gingivitis or sore throat. An infusion of sage can also relieve symptoms of excessive sweating and support memory. Its aromatic leaves lend themselves to herbal teas and gargling.

Lemon balm (Melissa officinalis)

Lemon balm is often referred to as the herb of calm. Its leaves with a delicate lemon aroma have sedative, antiviral and digestive properties. Lemon balm herbal tea is perfect for reducing anxiety, improving sleep and soothing stress-related gastrointestinal disorders. It is also useful for relieving the discomfort of chapped lips caused by herpes.

Ginger (Zingiber officinale)

Ginger is a root famous for its anti-inflammatory and digestive properties. An infusion of fresh ginger with lemon is a classic remedy for nausea, while its ability to improve circulation makes it useful for muscle and joint pain. Ginger can be used fresh, dried or as an oil.

Echinacea (Echinacea purpurea)

This plant is renowned for its ability to stimulate the immune system. Echinacea roots and leaves are used in herbal teas and tinctures to reduce the duration of cold and flu symptoms. It is an easy-to-grow perennial plant and valuable for the winter months.

Rosemary (Rosmarinus officinalis)

Rosemary is not only a culinary herb but also a powerful stimulant for the body and mind. It is rich in antioxidants, and its infusion can improve memory and mental energy. Rosemary essential oil is useful for relieving muscle aches and pains and promoting circulation. The plant is hardy and grows well in warm, sunny environments.

Yarrow (Achillea millefolium)

Yarrow is a versatile herb with anti-inflammatory and astringent properties. It is useful for treating wounds and abrasions, but also for relieving menstrual cramps and intestinal pain. Yarrow infusion is particularly effective for reducing fever and improving digestion.

Hypericum (Hypericum perforatum)

Hypericum is known as "St. John's Wort" and is famous for its antidepressant and antiseptic properties. It is used in the form of herbal teas to improve mood and as an oil to treat mild burns and skin irritations. Caution: St. John's Wort can interact with some medications, so it should be used with caution.

Fennel (Foeniculum vulgare)

Fennel is a valuable ally for the digestive tract. Fennel seeds, rich in essential oils, are often used in infusions to relieve bloating and colic. It is a perfect plant for the whole family, including children, because of its natural gentleness and sweetness.

Aloe Vera (Aloe barbadensis)

Aloe vera is one of the best-known medicinal plants in the world. The gel extracted from its leaves is used to soothe sunburns, moisturize the skin and treat minor irritations. Internally, aloe vera juice is useful for aiding digestion, but it should be used in moderation.

Dandelion (Taraxacum officinale)

Dandelion is a powerful natural depurative and diuretic. Its leaves and roots help support liver health and improve digestion. An infusion of dandelion root is ideal for those who want a natural detox, while fresh leaves can be added to salads.

Before you start working with herbs, it is important to consider some best practices:

- **Experiment with small amounts**: To better understand the effects and reduce the risk of waste.
- **Buy or grow organic herbs**: To ensure purity and effectiveness of remedies.
- **Keep an herbal journal**: Jotting down recipes, doses and personal reactions to remedies is an excellent way to build experience and knowledge.

Medicinal plants represent the heart of the home pharmacy. By starting with these indispensable herbs, beginners can develop a practical knowledge that will expand as they grow their experience and repertoire. Each plant offers a gateway to a greater awareness of nature's power and its healing possibilities.

LOCAL PLANTS VS. EXOTIC PLANTS: WHAT TO CHOOSE AND WHY

When it comes to building a home pharmacy, choosing between local and exotic plants is an important step. Each category has its advantages and limitations, and a balanced combination can ensure a versatile and sustainable pharmacy. Understanding the context of the plants you choose to use is essential not only for their effectiveness but also for the environmental and practical impact of their use.

LOCAL PLANTS: A LINK TO THE TERRITORY
Local plants are those that grow naturally in your environment or can be grown easily in your region. These plants offer several advantages, especially for those new to herbalism.

Advantages of Local Plants
1. **Ease of Access**: Local plants can be found in markets, nurseries, or even in the wild. For example, herbs such as rosemary, sage, and dandelion grow abundantly in Italy.
2. **Climate Adaptability**: Because they are already adapted to your environment, local plants require less care than exotic plants, which may need special conditions (e.g., specific temperatures, constant watering).
3. **Tradition and Local Knowledge**: Local plants have a long history of use in traditional medicine in your region. This means you can easily find recipes and methods of use that have been passed down through the ages.
4. **Sustainability**: Growing local plants reduces the environmental impact associated with importing exotic species and supports local biodiversity.

Examples of Local Plants
- Dandelion: Grows wild in meadows and gardens and is known for its depurative and digestive properties.
- Lavender: Common in Mediterranean regions, it is a versatile plant used for stress, insomnia and irritated skin.
- Rosemary: A hardy shrub that can also be easily grown in pots, useful for energizing herbal teas and stimulating massages.
- Chamomile: Known for generations, it is easy to grow and ideal for relaxing herbal teas.

EXOTIC PLANTS: THE ATTRACTION OF UNIQUENESS
Exotic plants come from other parts of the world and often carry with them an aura of mystery and novelty. Some of these plants, such as ginger or turmeric, have also become essential in Western medicine because of their powerful healing properties.

Benefits of Exotic Plants
1. **Unique Properties**: Many exotic plants contain active ingredients that are not commonly found in local plants. For example, ginger is known for its anti-inflammatory and warming effects.
2. **Versatility**: Some exotic plants, such as aloe vera, can be used for a wide range of problems, from irritated skin to digestion.
3. **Exposure to New Traditions**: Using exotic plants allows you to explore different herbal traditions, such as Ayurveda or Chinese medicine, enriching your knowledge and repertoire.

Challenges of Exotic Plants
- **Availability**: It is not always easy to obtain fresh exotic plants, and they often have to be purchased in dried or processed form.
- **High Costs**: Exotic plants can be more expensive than local plants, especially if imported.
- **Climate Adaptation**: Not all exotic plants adapt easily to the local climate, which may require greenhouses or spe-

cial care.

Examples of Exotic Plants
- **Ginger**: Native to Asia, it is a versatile plant used for nausea, inflammation and colds.
- **Aloe Vera**: A succulent plant native to warm regions, excellent for moisturizing and healing the skin.
- **Turmeric**: Known as "spice gold," it is an anti-inflammatory root used in herbal teas and ointments.
- **Echinacea**: Native to North America, it is popular for immune system support.

WHICH ONE TO CHOOSE?

Choosing between local and exotic plants depends on your goals, resources and level of experience. If you are just starting out, focusing on local plants is a sensible strategy. They are not only more accessible, but also allow you to develop a deeper connection with your natural environment. Once you gain experience, you can expand your pharmacy by including some exotic plants to expand your therapeutic possibilities.

Practical Example: Combining Local and Exotic

Suppose you want to create an herbal tea to improve digestion:
- Local base: Use mint and fennel, both plants that are easy to find and grow.
- Exotic touch: Add a slice of fresh ginger to enhance the effect and impart a spicy note.

This combination demonstrates how local and exotic plants can work together to create comprehensive and effective remedies.

Balancing local and exotic plants is a matter of practicality and personal preference. Deepening your knowledge of the plants around you will give you a solid starting point, while exploring exotic species will add a dimension of discovery and novelty to your herbal journey. By cultivating this duality, you can build a home pharmacy that is as efficient as it is rich in culture and tradition.

HERB IDENTIFICATION: TECHNIQUES FOR RECOGNIZING PLANTS IN NATURE AND DIFFERENCES BETWEEN SIMILAR SPECIES

One of the most fascinating aspects of herbalism is the ability to harvest plants directly from nature. However, this practice requires skill and care, as many plants may appear similar at first glance but differ significantly in their properties or even be toxic. The ability to correctly identify herbs is critical to ensure safety and efficacy in your remedies.

WHY IS HERB RECOGNITION IMPORTANT?
Picking herbs without proper identification can lead to dangerous mistakes. For example, some toxic plants, such as hemlock, resemble edible plants such as parsley or wild fennel. In addition, accurately identifying a plant allows you to take full advantage of its therapeutic properties. Each plant has distinctive characteristics that can be observed through careful study and experience.

BASIC IDENTIFICATION TECHNIQUES
To begin, it is helpful to know the basic botanical characteristics of plants, including leaf shape, flower type, scent and even where they grow. Here are some essential techniques for identifying herbs in the wild:

1. Observe the Shape of the Leaves
Leaves are one of the easiest features to examine. Pay attention to their shape (rounded, lanceolate, etc.), margin (smooth, serrated, serrated) and arrangement on the stem (opposite, alternate or spiral). For example, lemon balm and mint have similar leaves, but lemon balm has a more serrated margin and a lemony aroma.

2. Examine the Flowers

Flowers provide crucial information about a plant's identity. Look at the color, shape, number of petals and how they are arranged. Chamomile, for example, has white flowers with a prominent yellow center and a distinctive sweet scent that distinguishes it from daisy, which may look similar but does not have the same aroma.

3. Pay Attention to the Scent

Many medicinal herbs have a distinctive scent that makes them easily recognizable. Gently crush a leaf between your fingers and smell it: lavender has a calming floral aroma, while rosemary is pungent and stimulating. Scent can be a key criterion for distinguishing between similar-looking plants.

4. Study the Growth Environment

Plants often grow in specific environments, which can help you narrow down the possibilities. For example, wild thyme tends to thrive in dry, sunny soils, while horsetail prefers moist areas near waterways.

5. Consult Botanical Guides and Manuals

Carrying an illustrated guidebook with you is a great idea for identifying herbs in the field. These tools provide detailed descriptions and pictures to compare the plants you encounter. Many manuals also include details about harvest seasons and habitats.

DIFFERENCES BETWEEN SIMILAR PLANTS

Some plants may look identical at first glance, but they have subtle characteristics that distinguish them. Here are some examples of commonly confused plants:

Chamomile vs. Meadow Daisy

Chamomile has a sweet and relaxing scent, while the daisy does not give off the same aroma. Also, the petals of chamomile tend to bend downward with time, which is not the case with daisy.

Wild fennel vs. hemlock

Both have similar stems and feathery leaves, but wild fennel exudes a distinctive anise scent, while hemlock is odorless and highly toxic. In addition, fennel stems are smooth and green, while hemlock stems are often stained purple.

Lemon Balm vs. Dead White Nettle

Lemon balm has a lemony scent and smooth leaves, while white dead nettle does not have the same smell and is slightly hairy. Both grow in similar environments, but lemon balm is more suitable for medicinal use.

BEWARE OF TOXIC PLANTS

It is essential to remember that some plants can be toxic if harvested or used incorrectly. Learn to recognize dangerous species in your area, such as nightshade or oleander. Never pick a plant that you are not completely sure you can identify. When in doubt, consult an expert or qualified herbalist.

TOOLS TO FACILITATE IDENTIFICATION

As technology advances, there are now plant recognition apps that can help you quickly identify a species. Apps such as PlantNet or PictureThis allow you to take a photo and compare it to a botanical database. Although useful, these tools should be used in conjunction with basic knowledge and reliable guides.

Herb identification requires practice, patience, and a keen eye for detail. Developing this skill will allow you not only to collect plants safely but also to deepen your connection with nature. With time and experience, plant recognition will become second nature, allowing you to continually expand your home pharmacy with confidence and competence.

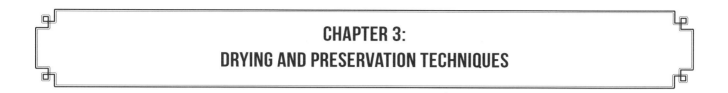

CHAPTER 3:
DRYING AND PRESERVATION TECHNIQUES

METHODS FOR DRYING HERBS - TRADITIONAL AND MODERN

Drying herbs is an art that has its roots in the oldest traditions, but today can be enhanced by modern tools. This technique is essential for preserving the effectiveness of the active ingredients contained in plants, keeping their aromatic, medicinal and nutritional properties intact. Choosing the right method depends on both the resources available and the type of plant you wish to preserve.

The traditional air-drying method is, without a doubt, the most natural and accessible. It is a practice that requires patience, but offers extraordinary results when done correctly. Begin by harvesting the herbs at the right time, usually in the early morning hours when the essential oil in the leaves is at its peak and the moisture of the night has dissipated. Herbs should be handled gently to avoid damaging delicate parts such as flowers and leaves. Once harvested, tying small bunches with natural twine is the next step. Each bunch should be tight enough to hold the stems together, but not too tight, to allow air to circulate freely.

Air drying requires a dry, shady, well-ventilated space. Exposure to direct sunlight is detrimental, as it degrades the active ingredients and alters the color of the plants. A well-ventilated attic, shed or quiet corner of the house can be perfect for hanging bunches upside down. Drying can take one to three weeks, depending on the climate and the thickness of the plants. To tell if the herb is ready, just try snapping a stem: if it breaks with a sharp sound, it is dried properly.

A more modern approach involves the use of dryers. These devices are designed to dry plants precisely by controlling temperature and airflow. The use of a dryer eliminates uncertainties related to weather conditions and significantly reduces the time needed to complete the process. After harvesting, the herbs are spread evenly on the dryer trays, taking care not to overlap them. The ideal temperature ranges between 35 and 40 degrees Celsius, a range gentle enough to preserve the herbs' medicinal and aromatic properties. The advantage of this method is the consistency of the result: each leaf, flower or stem will be dried evenly.

Modern drying, however, is not without its challenges. It is important not to set temperatures too high, as they can "cook" the herbs, compromising their qualities. Also, although it is a quick option, it does not offer the same nostalgic and natural appeal as the traditional method. However, for those who live in humid environments or have limited space, the dryer is a practical and reliable solution.

Whether you choose the traditional or modern method, the quality of the drying always depends on how you treat the plants from the moment of harvest until the process is complete. Every leaf and flower retains some of its healing power, a little treasure of nature that you can use for months to come. Drying is more than just a practical step: it is a ritual, a direct link to the long history of herbalism.

HOW TO PRESERVE OILS, TINCTURES AND HERBAL TEAS WITHOUT LOSING EFFICACY

Preservation of herbal preparations is a crucial step in keeping their therapeutic benefits intact over time. Oils, tinctures and herbal teas require specific care to preserve their properties, avoiding deterioration due to light, heat and oxygen. Learning how to properly store these preparations means ensuring that your efforts in extracting and processing plants do not go to waste, while providing a home pharmacy ready for every need.

Infused oils, often used for topical purposes, require special attention to protection from light and air. After infusing the herb in a carrier oil, such as olive or almond oil, it is critical to filter the liquid thoroughly to remove all traces of plant material. Even a small residue can degrade the oil, causing unpleasant odors and loss of effectiveness. Once filtered, the oil should be decanted into dark glass bottles that protect it from direct light and stored in a cool, dry place. The refrigerator is a good option, especially in hot climates, but for oils that tend to solidify at low temperatures, such as coconut oil, a cool cabinet may be sufficient. Well-stored infused oils can last up to a year.

Tinctures, by their nature, are more stable than oils due to the presence of alcohol or vinegar used as solvents. Once prepared, a tincture can last several years as long as it is stored properly. Again, dark glass is the best ally, as it reduces exposure to light, which could degrade the active compounds. Dropper bottles are ideal not only for storage, but also for accurate dosing. Tinctures should be kept away from heat sources and preferably in an airtight cabinet. Remember to always label bottles with the name of the herb, the solvent used and the date of preparation so you know exactly what you are using and how long it has been stored.

Herbal teas and infusions, being water-based preparations, are by their nature less durable and should be consumed within a few hours of preparation to take full advantage of their properties. However, if you need to store them for a short time, transferring the herbal tea to an airtight container and refrigerating it immediately is the best choice. A refrigerated herbal tea can last up to 24 hours, but it is important to warm it gently before consumption, avoiding high temperatures that could compromise the active ingredients.

To prolong the shelf life of herbal tea ingredients, however, it is essential to store dried herbs properly. Glass jars with airtight closures are ideal, as they protect against moisture and air, the main enemies of dried plants. Again, dark glass is preferable, but if you only have clear jars, they can be stored in a cupboard away from light. Adding a small bag of food-grade silica gel to the jar can help keep moisture to a minimum. When possible, store each herb separately to avoid odor or flavor contamination.

A final item to consider for all preparations is monitoring their quality over time. Rancid oils, faded tinctures, or herbs lacking aroma are obvious signs that the product is no longer effective. Taking an organized approach to storage, with clearly visible labels and regular checks, ensures that your home pharmacy will always remain a reliable wellness ally.

Careful storage is not just a useful practice, but a gesture of respect for the plants and the work you have put into processing them. Each jar or bottle represents a little treasure chest of health and nature, ready to support you and your loved ones safely and effectively.

AVOIDING MOLD AND SPOILAGE-COMMON MISTAKES TO AVOID

One of the biggest challenges in preserving medicinal herbs is preventing mold, spoilage and loss of potency. The appearance of mold not only renders the preparation unusable, but can be hazardous to health. Understanding the factors that cause these problems and adopting strategies to avoid them is essential for a safe and durable home pharmacy.

The first common mistake is harvesting herbs at the wrong times of day or in unsuitable weather conditions. Plants harvested during the hottest hours, when humidity is still high, retain too much water in the tissues, making drying more difficult and increasing the risk of mold. Harvesting should take place early in the morning, after the dew has dried but before the sun becomes too intense. It is equally important to avoid harvesting wet plants from rain or irrigation, as excess water can become trapped during the drying process.

Another frequent mistake is not giving herbs the space they need during drying. When plants are hung too close together or crammed into a dryer, air cannot circulate freely. This lack of ventilation creates a favorable environment for mold development. Hanging small bunches or distributing herbs in thin layers on drying trays ensures that air reaches every part of the plants. In a dryer, it is critical not to overload the trays and to check that the airflow remains even.

Haste is often the enemy of quality. Many people stop the drying process too early, storing herbs that are not completely dry. Even minimal residual moisture can lead to mold growth once herbs are stored in airtight jars or bags. To check that an herb is completely dried, try breaking a stem: if it bends without breaking, the process is not yet finished.

During storage, ambient humidity is another critical factor. Jars that do not seal properly or are opened frequently in humid environments can absorb moisture from the air, promoting spoilage. Storing herbs in airtight containers and in a cool, dry place away from the kitchen or bathroom is best. If you live in an area with high humidity, you can add a small bag of food-grade silica gel to the jars to absorb excess moisture.

As for oils and dyes, using unsterilized tools is a common mistake that compromises the durability of preparations. Contaminants such as bacteria and microscopic molds can introduce themselves during decanting or filtering, leading to deterioration even under optimal storage conditions. Before handling oils or tinctures, make sure everything-from jars to spoons-is perfectly clean and dry. In the case of infused oils, check that no plant residues remain in the liquid, as these can ferment or mold over time.

An often underestimated mistake is exposure to direct sunlight. Although herbs seem well preserved in clear jars, light quickly degrades the active ingredients, reducing the effectiveness of the product. Using dark glass jars or storing preparations in a dark cabinet is a simple but effective solution.

Finally, lack of labeling and monitoring is a mistake that can lead to using expired or deteriorated products. Each jar, bottle, or bag should be labeled with the contents, the date of preparation, and, if possible, the estimated expiration date. A useful rule of thumb is to check stocks regularly, looking for signs of spoilage such as unpleasant odors, altered colors or unusual textures.

Avoiding mold and spoilage requires attention to detail and some discipline, but the results are worth the effort. Storing medicinal herbs with care means being able to rely on them in times of need, knowing that they are safe, potent and ready for use. This level of dedication not only elevates the quality of your home pharmacy, it also strengthens your connection to the natural world and your respect for the gifts it gives us.

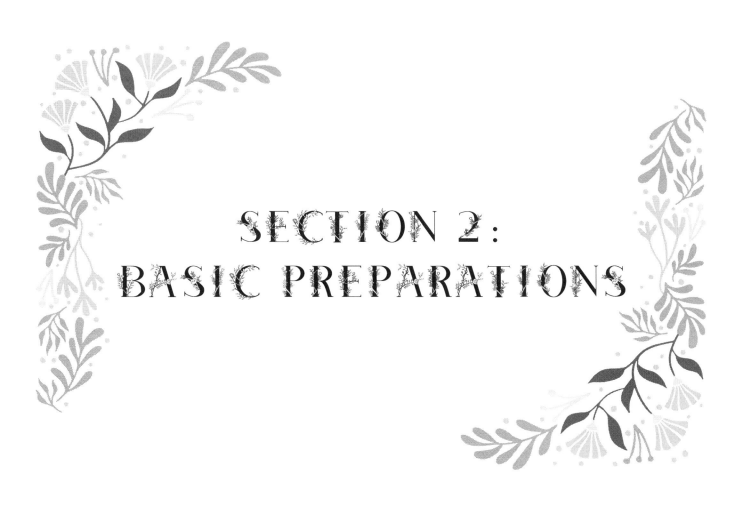

SECTION 2:
BASIC PREPARATIONS

CHAPTER 4:
TINCTURES AND EXTRACTS — THE MAGIC OF MACERATION

WHAT IS A TINCTURE? HOW DOES IT WORK AND WHICH SOLVENTS TO USE

Tinctures represent one of the oldest and most versatile methods of extracting and preserving the active ingredients of medicinal plants. These are liquid preparations obtained by steeping plant parts in a solvent, usually alcohol, for an extended period. This process allows the beneficial chemical compounds of the herbs to be captured in a highly concentrated and easy-to-use form. Tinctures are distinguished by their efficacy because the active ingredients are quickly made available to the body, often more directly than herbal teas or decoctions.

But what makes a tincture so special? The answer lies in the process itself. During maceration, the solvent penetrates the plant tissues, dissolving and drawing out the water- and fat-soluble compounds present. This mechanism preserves not only the aromas and flavors, but more importantly the medicinal properties of the plants, making them stable and usable for months or even years. A well-made tincture becomes a kind of "preserve" of health, ready to be used with just a few drops as needed.

The choice of solvent is one of the most crucial aspects in preparing a tincture. Traditionally, alcohol has been considered the ideal solvent because of its ability to extract a wide spectrum of compounds, from tannins to terpenes to alkaloids and flavonoids. In addition, alcohol acts as a natural preservative, preventing the development of mold and bacteria. The alcohol content to be used varies depending on the type of plant and the active ingredients to be extracted. For example, for herbs with milder principles, such as chamomile, lighter alcohol is preferable, while stronger alcohols are used for plants with stronger compounds, such as St. John's Wort or echinacea root.

However, alcohol is not the only possible solvent. Alternatively, vegetable glycerin or vinegar can be used, making tinctures accessible even to those who prefer to avoid using alcohol. Glycerin, with its sweet taste and viscous texture, is ideal for children and sensitive people, although its extraction capacity is less than that of alcohol. Vinegar, on the other hand, offers a dual function: extraction and digestive support. The choice of solvent often depends on the intended use of the dye and personal preference, but it is important to understand that each solvent has its own limitations and advantages, and their use requires awareness and precision.

The quality of the tincture also depends on the ratio of plant to solvent, known as the "weight ratio." This ratio varies depending on the plant used and the desired intensity of the dye. For example, a standard ratio of 1:5 means that for every part of dry plant, five parts of solvent are used. This balance ensures that the tincture is concentrated enough to be effective, but not so dense that it overloads the body or is impractical to use.

Another fascinating aspect of tinctures is their ability to adapt to individual needs. Custom blends can be created by combining several plants in one solution to achieve specific synergies. For example, a combined tincture of echinacea, ginger, and elderberry can become an ideal remedy to support the immune system during the cold season.

Preparing a tincture takes time and patience, but the result repays the effort. After steeping, which can last from two to six weeks, the liquid is filtered and transferred to dark glass bottles to protect it from light and preserve its properties. Each drop represents a concentrate of nature's wisdom, encapsulated in a solution that is easy to dose and extraordinarily effective.

In conclusion, tincture is not only a natural remedy, but a symbol of the connection between human beings and the plant world. It is a bridge that unites tradition and modernity, offering a practical and powerful means of bringing the benefits of plants into daily life. The choice of solvent, preparation, and proper use make the difference between a simple extract and a remedy that can truly support health and well-being.

To dilute food alcohol to 95 percent and get the correct alcohol content for your preparations, it is important to use only quality water, preferably demineralized or distilled water. Follow these steps:

1. PROPORTION FOR DILUTION

To obtain a specific alcohol concentration, use the following formula:

$$V_1 \times C_1 = V_2 \times C_2$$

Where:

- V_1: initial volume of 95% alcohol.
- C_1: initial concentration (95%).
- V_2: desired final volume.
- C_2: desired final concentration.

Example: To obtain 1 liter of 40% alcohol from 95% alcohol, calculate:

$$V_1 = \frac{V_2 \times C_2}{C_1} = \frac{1000 \times 40}{95} \approx 421 \, \text{ml.}$$

You will need 421 ml of alcohol and 579 ml of water.

2. PROCEDURE

Always pour the alcohol into the water (never the other way around!) to avoid unwanted thermal reactions. Stir slowly and let the mixture sit for a few hours or days so that any reactions settle.

3. WATER QUALITY.

Use distilled or demineralized water, which is free of minerals and impurities. This prevents unwanted flavors from transferring to the mixture.

4. STORAGE

Store diluted alcohol in tightly sealed glass containers in a cool place away from direct light. In this way, you will dilute the alcohol without compromising its flavor or quality.

BASIC RECIPES — ECHINACEA TINCTURE, VALERIAN TINCTURE, AND MORE

Basic recipes for making tinctures are the starting point for any home pharmacy enthusiast. Each tincture encapsulates the healing power of a plant in a concentrated and easily usable form. Here we present some of the most common and effective tinctures, explaining how to make them step by step. These preparations are not only useful for dealing with a variety of ailments, but also offer a practical and rewarding experience that connects you directly with nature.

TINCTURE OF ECHINACEA

Botanical Description: Echinacea (Echinacea purpurea or Echinacea angustifolia) is a perennial plant belonging to the Asteraceae family. Native to North America, it is characterized by daisy-like flowers with pinkish-purple petals and a prominent central cone.

Properties: Echinacea is known for its immune-stimulating, antiviral and anti-inflammatory properties. It is mainly used to prevent and treat colds, flu and respiratory tract infections.

Ingredients:
- 100 g dried echinacea root (or 200 g if fresh).
- 500 ml of 70° alcohol (vodka or diluted food alcohol).

Preparation:
1. Clean and cut the echinacea root into small pieces.
2. Place the root in a sterilized glass jar and fill it three-quarters full.
3. Cover with alcohol, making sure the root is completely submerged.
4. Seal the jar and store in a cool, dark place for 4 to 6 weeks, shaking daily.
5. Filter with gauze and transfer the liquid into dark glass bottles.

Dosage: 20-30 drops diluted in water, 2-3 times daily at the first signs of a cold.
Precautions: Avoid in case of allergy to Asteraceae. Prolonged use (more than 8 weeks) is not recommended.

VALERIAN TINCTURE

Botanical Description: Valerian (Valeriana officinalis) is an herbaceous perennial plant belonging to the Caprifoliaceae family. It grows in moist, temperate areas, characterized by erect stems and compound leaves, as well as small white or pink flowers.

Properties: Valerian is celebrated for its sedative, anxiolytic and relaxing properties. It is commonly used to relieve stress, insomnia and states of nervous tension.

Ingredients:
- 100 g dried valerian root.
- 500 ml of 40° alcohol (vodka or brandy).

Preparation:
1. Reduce the valerian root into small pieces.
2. Place the root in a clean glass jar, filling half the container.
3. Add the alcohol until the plant is completely covered.
4. Seal and let macerate in a dark place for 4 to 6 weeks, shaking daily.
5. Strain and transfer to dark glass bottles.

Dosage: 10-20 drops diluted in water before bedtime or during anxious situations.
Precautions: Avoid excessive or combined use with sedatives. May cause drowsiness.

TINCTURE OF CALENDULA

Botanical Description: Marigold (Calendula officinalis), also known as "flowering marigold," is an annual or perennial herbaceous plant in the Asteraceae family. It is distinguished by its vibrant orange or yellow flowers, often used for both ornamental and medicinal purposes. It is native to southern Europe but cultivated widely throughout the world.

Properties: Calendula is renowned for its anti-inflammatory, antiseptic and healing properties. It is often used to treat skin problems, such as irritation, wounds and acne, and as an aid in inflammation of the digestive tract.

Ingredients:
- 100 g dried marigold flowers.
- 500 ml of 70° alcohol or apple cider vinegar for an alcohol-free version.

Preparation:
1. Harvest the calendula flowers, making sure they are completely dry before using them.
2. Place the flowers in a glass jar, filling it halfway.
3. Pour in the alcohol or apple cider vinegar until the flowers are completely covered.
4. Seal the jar and store it in a cool, dark place for 4 weeks, shaking daily.
5. Filter with gauze and transfer the liquid to dark glass bottles with dropper caps.

Dosage: For external use, dilute a few drops in water and apply with a cotton ball. For internal use, if prepared with alcohol, take 10-15 drops diluted in water to relieve inflammation of the digestive tract.
Precautions: Do not apply to open wounds without consulting an expert. Avoid in case of allergy to Asteraceae.

PEPPERMINT TINCTURE

Botanical Description: Peppermint (Mentha × piperita) is a natural hybrid of water mint and spearmint. It is a perennial plant in the Lamiaceae family, with deep green lanceolate leaves and small purplish flowers. It grows rapidly in temperate and humid climates.

Properties: Peppermint is valued for its refreshing, digestive and antispasmodic properties. It is ideal for relieving digestive disorders, nausea, headaches and nasal congestion.

Ingredients:
- 100 g dried or fresh peppermint leaves.
- 500 ml of 40° alcohol (vodka or brandy).

Preparation:
1. Wash the fresh leaves thoroughly, if used, and dry them.
2. Place the leaves in a clean glass jar, filling half the container.
3. Add the alcohol, making sure all the leaves are submerged.
4. Seal the jar and store it in a cool, dark place for 3-4 weeks, shaking it daily.
5. Filter with gauze and decant the liquid into dark glass bottles.

Dosage: Take 10-15 drops diluted in water after meals to relieve digestive disorders or apply externally to massage on temples for headaches.
Precautions: Avoid high doses in people with gastroesophageal reflux, as it can worsen symptoms.

TINCTURE OF HYPERICUM

Botanical Description: Hypericum (Hypericum perforatum), also known as "St. John's Wort," is an herbaceous perennial plant in the Hypericaceae family. It is distinguished by its bright yellow flowers with tiny perforations visible on the leaves, which contain glands filled with essential oil. It grows wild in sunny meadows and fields.

Properties: St. John's Wort is famous for its antidepressant, anti-inflammatory and healing properties. It is used to improve mood in mild states of depression, treat anxiety disorders and soothe skin wounds.

Ingredients:
- 100 g fresh St. John's Wort flowers (or 50 g dried).
- 500 ml of 70° alcohol (vodka or diluted food alcohol).

Preparation:
1. Pick the fresh flowers in full bloom, preferably in the morning, when they are rich in essential oils.
2. Place the flowers in a clean glass jar, filling it halfway.
3. Cover the flowers completely with alcohol, stirring gently to remove any air bubbles.
4. Seal the jar tightly and store it in a dark, cool place for 4 to 6 weeks, shaking the container daily.
5. Strain with gauze and transfer the liquid to dark glass bottles.

Dosage: 10-20 drops diluted in water, 2-3 times daily, to improve mood or soothe anxious states. For external use, apply to wounds or light burns.

Precautions: St. John's Wort may interact with many medications, including antidepressants and oral contraceptives. Consult a physician before use.

THYME TINCTURE

Botanical Description: Thyme (Thymus vulgaris) is an aromatic perennial plant in the Lamiaceae family. It is characterized by small woody stems, narrow aromatic leaves, and pale purple flowers. It grows wild in dry, sunny soils and is widely cultivated for culinary and medicinal use.

Properties: Thyme is known for its antiseptic, antibacterial and anti-inflammatory properties. It is an excellent remedy for respiratory infections, coughs and digestive problems.

Ingredients:
- 100 g dried thyme leaves and flowers.
- 500 ml of 40° alcohol (vodka or brandy).

Preparation:
1. Harvest thyme leaves and flowers during full bloom.
2. Place the thyme in a clean glass jar, filling it halfway.
3. Pour in the alcohol until the plant parts are completely covered. Stir gently.
4. Seal the jar and store it in a cool, dark place for 3-4 weeks, shaking the container daily.
5. Strain with gauze and transfer the liquid into dark glass bottles.

Dosage: 10-20 drops diluted in water, up to 3 times a day, to relieve coughs and congestion or support digestion.

Precautions: Avoid if you have an allergy to the Lamiaceae family. Do not use in large doses during pregnancy.

TINCTURE OF CHAMOMILE

Botanical Description: Chamomile (Matricaria chamomilla) is an annual herbaceous plant belonging to the Asteraceae family. It is characterized by small daisy-like flowers with white petals and a central yellow disk. Native to Europe, it is widely cultivated for its medicinal and aromatic properties.

Properties: Chamomile is celebrated for its calming, antispasmodic and digestive properties. It is used to relieve stress, insomnia and digestive problems such as colic or abdominal cramps.

Ingredients:
- 100 g dried chamomile flowers.
- 500 ml of 40° alcohol (vodka or brandy).

Preparation:
1. Harvest the chamomile flowers and dry them completely if using fresh ones.
2. Place the flowers in a clean glass jar, filling it halfway.
3. Add the alcohol until the flowers are completely covered. Stir gently to remove any air bubbles.
4. Seal the jar and store it in a cool, dark place for 3 to 4 weeks, shaking it daily.
5. Filter with gauze and transfer the liquid to dark glass bottles with dropper caps.

Dosage: 15-20 drops diluted in water or tea before bedtime to promote sleep or after meals to support digestion.
Precautions: Avoid if you have an allergy to Asteraceae.

TINCTURE OF SAGE

Botanical Description: Sage (Salvia officinalis) is a perennial plant in the Lamiaceae family, with silvery-green lanceolate leaves and blue-purple flowers. It is native to the Mediterranean and known for its intense aroma and medicinal applications.

Properties: Sage is known for its antiseptic, digestive and hormone-regulating properties. It is often used for digestive disorders, mouth and throat infections, and to relieve menopausal symptoms.

Ingredients:
- 100 g dried sage leaves.
- 500 ml of 40° alcohol (vodka or brandy).

Preparation:
1. Break up the sage leaves to aid extraction.
2. Place them in a sterilized glass jar, filling half the container.
3. Pour in the alcohol until the leaves are completely covered.
4. Seal the jar and store in a dark place for 4 weeks, shaking it daily.
5. Strain and transfer to dark glass bottles.

Dosage: 10-15 drops diluted in water for digestive disorders or 20 drops for gargling in case of throat infections.
Precautions: Avoid prolonged use or in large doses during pregnancy.

GINGER TINCTURE

Botanical Description: Ginger (Zingiber officinale) is a perennial herbaceous plant native to tropical Asia, belonging to the Zingiberaceae family. The part used is the rhizome, which is gnarled, aromatic and yellowish inside.

Properties: Ginger is famous for its anti-inflammatory, digestive and stimulant properties. It is used to relieve nausea, improve digestion and support circulation.

Ingredients:
- 100 g fresh ginger rhizome.
- 500 ml of 40° alcohol (vodka or brandy).

Preparation:
1. Wash and peel the ginger rhizome, then cut it into thin slices.
2. Place the rhizome in a sterilized glass jar, filling it three-quarters full.
3. Cover with alcohol, making sure all slices are submerged.
4. Seal and store in a cool, dark place for 3-4 weeks, shaking daily.
5. Strain with gauze and transfer the liquid to dark glass bottles.

Dosage: 10-20 drops diluted in water or tea to relieve nausea or improve digestion.
Precautions: Avoid if you have stomach ulcers or gastroesophageal reflux.

ROSEMARY TINCTURE

Botanical Description: Rosemary (Rosmarinus officinalis) is an evergreen shrub belonging to the Lamiaceae family. It is native to the Mediterranean and is characterized by fragrant green needle-shaped leaves with small blue or light purple flowers.

Properties: Rosemary is known for its stimulant, antioxidant and antiseptic properties. It is often used to improve circulation, stimulate memory, and treat digestive problems or muscle aches.

Ingredients:
- 100 g fresh rosemary leaves or 50 g dried leaves.
- 500 ml of 40° alcohol (vodka or brandy).

Preparation:
1. Wash and dry the fresh leaves, if used.
2. Place the leaves in a sterilized glass jar, filling half the container.
3. Cover with alcohol, making sure all the leaves are submerged.
4. Seal the jar and store it in a cool, dark place for 4 weeks, shaking it daily.
5. Filter the contents with gauze and transfer the liquid into dark glass bottles with dropper caps.

Dosage: 10-20 drops diluted in water or tea, once or twice a day, to stimulate concentration or improve digestion.
Precautions: Avoid in cases of pregnancy or uncontrolled hypertension.

LAVENDER TINCTURE

Botanical Description: Lavender (Lavandula angustifolia) is a perennial shrub in the Lamiaceae family, characterized by fragrant purple flowers growing on long stems and narrow greenish-gray leaves. Native to the Mediterranean, it is known for its calming scent and therapeutic properties.

Properties: Lavender is known for its relaxing, antispasmodic and antiseptic properties. It is used to relieve stress, insomnia, muscle tension and skin irritation.

Ingredients:
- 100 g dried lavender flowers.
- 500 ml of 40° alcohol (vodka or brandy).

Preparation:
1. Place the lavender flowers in a sterilized glass jar, filling it halfway.
2. Pour in the alcohol until the flowers are completely covered.
3. Seal the jar and store it in a cool, dark place for 4 weeks, shaking daily.
4. Filter with gauze and transfer the liquid to dark glass bottles.

Dosage: 10-20 drops diluted in water or tea before bedtime to promote sleep, or apply externally to relieve muscle aches.

Precautions: Avoid overuse if you suffer from hypotension.

FENNEL TINCTURE

Botanical Description: Fennel (Foeniculum vulgare) is a perennial herbaceous plant belonging to the Apiaceae family. It is characterized by hollow stems, feathery leaves and yellow umbrella-shaped flowers. Its characteristic aroma is due to the essential oils contained in the seeds.

Properties: Fennel is known for its digestive, antispasmodic and carminative properties. It is used to relieve digestive problems, bloating and colic.

Ingredients:
- 100 g dried fennel seeds.
- 500 ml of 40° alcohol (vodka or brandy).

Preparation:
1. Lightly crush the fennel seeds to release the essential oils.
2. Place the seeds in a sterilized glass jar, filling it halfway.
3. Pour in the alcohol until the seeds are completely covered.
4. Seal the jar and store it in a cool, dark place for 3 to 4 weeks, shaking daily.
5. Strain and transfer the liquid into dark glass bottles.

Dosage: 10-15 drops diluted in water after meals to aid digestion.

Precautions: Avoid if you have an allergy to Apiaceae.

TINCTURE OF LAUREL

Botanical Description: Laurel (Laurus nobilis) is an evergreen shrub belonging to the Lauraceae family. It is characterized by leathery, aromatic dark green leaves and small yellow flowers. Native to the Mediterranean, bay laurel is used both as a spice and as a medicinal remedy.

Properties: Laurel is known for its digestive, antiseptic and anti-inflammatory properties. It is especially useful for relieving indigestion, bloating and muscle aches.

Ingredients:
- 50 g fresh bay leaves (or 30 g dried).
- 500 ml of 40° alcohol (vodka or brandy).

Preparation:
1. Wash and dry the fresh bay leaves.
2. Lightly crush the leaves to help extract the essential oils.
3. Place the leaves in a sterilized glass jar, filling it one-third full.
4. Pour in the alcohol until the leaves are completely covered.
5. Seal the jar and store it in a cool, dark place for 4 weeks, shaking it daily.
6. Strain the liquid with gauze and transfer to dark glass bottles with dropper caps.

Dosage: 10-15 drops diluted in water after meals to aid digestion, or apply externally on muscle aches and pains.
Precautions: Avoid excessive dosages. Do not use during pregnancy without consulting an expert.

TINCTURE OF NETTLE

Botanical Description: Nettle (Urtica dioica) is an herbaceous perennial plant belonging to the Urticaceae family. It is distinguished by its quadrangular stems, serrated green leaves and urticating hairs that cover the entire plant.

Properties: Nettle is rich in minerals and vitamins, with diuretic, depurative and anti-inflammatory properties. It is used to treat arthritis, water retention and anemia.

Ingredients:
- 100 g fresh nettle leaves (or 50 g dried).
- 500 ml of 40° alcohol (vodka or brandy).

Preparation:
1. Harvest the nettle leaves with gloves to avoid irritation.
2. Place the leaves in a sterilized glass jar, filling it halfway.
3. Pour the alcohol over the leaves, making sure they are completely submerged.
4. Seal the jar and store it in a cool, dark place for 3-4 weeks, shaking it every day.
5. Strain with gauze and transfer the liquid to dark glass bottles.

Dosage: 15-20 drops diluted in water, 2-3 times a day, to support metabolism and improve circulation.
Precautions: Avoid in renal insufficiency or during pregnancy.

LEMON BALM TINCTURE

Botanical Description: Lemon balm (Melissa officinalis) is a perennial herbaceous plant belonging to the Lamiaceae family. It is characterized by its green, oval, toothed leaves, which give off a fresh lemon-like scent. Native to the Mediterranean, it is highly valued for its therapeutic properties.

Properties: Lemon balm is known for its calming, antispasmodic and digestive properties. It is ideal for relieving stress, anxiety, insomnia and gastrointestinal disorders such as bloating and cramping.

Ingredients:
- 100 g fresh lemon balm leaves (or 50 g dried).
- 500 ml of 40° alcohol (vodka or brandy).

Preparation:
1. Wash the fresh lemon balm leaves and dry them thoroughly.
2. Place the leaves in a sterilized glass jar, filling it halfway.
3. Pour the alcohol over the leaves, making sure they are completely covered.
4. Seal the jar and store it in a cool, dark place for 4 weeks, shaking the container daily.
5. Filter the contents with gauze and transfer the liquid to dark glass bottles.

Dosage: 10-20 drops diluted in water, 2-3 times daily, to relieve anxiety or aid digestion.
Precautions: Avoid high doses during pregnancy or if you have hypothyroidism.

TINCTURE OF HAWTHORN

Botanical Description: Hawthorn (Crataegus monogyna) is a thorny shrub belonging to the Rosaceae family. It is characterized by lobed leaves, white flowers and red berries. It is commonly found in Europe and is widely used in herbal medicine.

Properties: Hawthorn is valued for its cardioprotective, calming and hypotensive properties. It is used to regulate blood pressure, improve circulation and relieve anxiety.

Ingredients:
- 50 g fresh hawthorn flowers and leaves (or 30 g dried).
- 500 ml of 40° alcohol (vodka or brandy).

Preparation:
1. Harvest the hawthorn flowers and leaves during full bloom.
2. Place them in a sterilized glass jar, filling half the container.
3. Cover with alcohol until the plant parts are completely submerged.
4. Seal the jar and store in a cool, dark place for 3-4 weeks, shaking daily.
5. Strain with gauze and transfer the liquid into dark glass bottles.

Dosage: 15-20 drops diluted in water, 2-3 times daily, to support heart health or relieve anxiety.
Precautions: Avoid when taking heart medications without consulting a doctor.

DANDELION TINCTURE

Botanical Description: Dandelion (Taraxacum officinale) is an herbaceous perennial plant belonging to the Asteraceae family. It is characterized by toothed leaves, bright yellow flowers and feathery seeds that disperse in the wind. It is commonly found in meadows and fallow land around the world.

Properties: Dandelion is valued for its depurative, diuretic and digestive properties. It is used to support liver health, stimulate digestion and promote the elimination of excess fluids.

Ingredients:
- 100 g fresh dandelion roots (or 50 g dried).
- 500 ml of 40° alcohol (vodka or brandy).

Preparation:
1. Wash the fresh dandelion roots thoroughly and cut them into small pieces.
2. Place them in a sterilized glass jar, filling half the container.
3. Pour the alcohol over the roots, making sure they are completely submerged.
4. Seal the jar and store in a cool, dark place for 4 weeks, shaking daily.
5. Strain the liquid with gauze and transfer to dark glass bottles.

Dosage: 10-15 drops diluted in water, 2-3 times daily, to support digestion and promote purification.
Precautions: Avoid in case of gallstones or biliary obstruction.

JUNIPER TINCTURE

Botanical Description: Juniper (Juniperus communis) is an evergreen shrub in the Cupressaceae family. It is characterized by pointed needles and dark blue or black berries, which are used in both cooking and phytotherapy. It commonly grows in Europe, Asia and North America.

Properties: Juniper is known for its diuretic, antiseptic and digestive properties. It is used to promote fluid elimination, relieve urinary tract infections and improve digestion.

Ingredients:
- 50 g fresh juniper berries or 30 g dried.
- 500 ml of 40° alcohol (vodka or brandy).

Preparation:
1. Lightly crush the juniper berries to release the essential oils.
2. Place the berries in a sterilized glass jar, filling it one-third full.
3. Pour the alcohol over the berries, making sure they are completely submerged.
4. Seal the jar and store it in a cool, dark place for 3-4 weeks, shaking it daily.
5. Strain the liquid with gauze and transfer to dark glass bottles.

Dosage: 10-15 drops diluted in water, up to 2 times a day, to promote diuresis and improve digestion.
Precautions: Avoid in renal insufficiency or during pregnancy.

TINCTURE OF ALOE VERA

Botanical Description: Aloe vera (Aloe barbadensis) is a succulent plant belonging to the Asphodelaceae family. It is characterized by fleshy, spiny leaves containing a transparent gel rich in active ingredients. Native to North Africa, it is widely cultivated worldwide for its healing properties.

Properties: Aloe vera is known for its healing, moisturizing and anti-inflammatory properties. It is used both for internal use as digestive and immune support and for external use to soothe skin irritations and burns.

Ingredients:
- 100 g fresh gel extracted from aloe vera leaves.
- 500 ml of 70° alcohol (vodka or diluted food alcohol).

Preparation:
1. Harvest one or two ripe aloe vera leaves from the base of the plant.
2. Wash the leaves thoroughly and remove the outer skin to extract the clear gel.
3. Place the gel in a sterilized glass jar.
4. Pour the alcohol over the gel, making sure it is completely submerged.
5. Seal the jar and store in a cool, dark place for 2-3 weeks, shaking daily.
6. Strain the liquid through a gauze or fine mesh filter and transfer the tincture to dark glass bottles with dropper caps.

Dosage:
For internal use: 5-10 drops diluted in water or juice, 1-2 times daily, to aid digestion and improve immune function.
For external use: Apply a few drops directly to minor wounds, burns or skin irritations.

Precautions: Avoid internal use if you are pregnant, nursing or have kidney problems. External use is generally safe, but test a small area of skin for allergic reactions.

TINCTURE OF EUCALYPTUS

Botanical Description: Eucalyptus (Eucalyptus globulus) is an evergreen tree in the Myrtaceae family, native to Australia. It is distinguished by its long, aromatic leaves, which release a fresh, balsamic scent.

Properties: Eucalyptus is known for its expectorant, antiseptic and cooling properties. It is used to relieve symptoms of colds, coughs and nasal congestion.

Ingredients:
- 50 g of dried eucalyptus leaves.
- 500 ml of 70° alcohol (vodka or diluted food grade alcohol).

Preparation:
1. Crush the dried leaves and place them in a sterilized glass jar, filling it halfway.
2. Pour the alcohol over the leaves, making sure they are completely submerged.
3. Seal the jar and store in a cool, dark place for 3 weeks, shaking it daily.
4. Filter the contents with gauze and transfer the liquid to dark glass bottles with dropper caps.

Dosage:
For internal use: 10 drops diluted in water or hot tea, 1-2 times daily, to support breathing.
For external use: Add a few drops to a carrier oil and apply to the chest to relieve congestion.

Precautions: Do not use during pregnancy or for children under 12 years of age without consulting a physician.

HOW TO DOSE – PRECISE CALCULATIONS FOR SAFE ADMINISTRATION

A tincture is a highly concentrated natural remedy, and the correct dosage is critical to ensure the safety and efficacy of the treatment. The dosage approach varies depending on the plant used, the condition to be treated, and the individual characteristics of the person taking it, such as age, weight, and general health status. Below, we explore the basic principles and practical calculations for safe dosing.

FACTORS TO CONSIDER FOR DOSAGE
1. **Concentration of Tincture**: The concentration of the tincture depends on the weight ratio of plant to solvent (e.g., 1:5 means that 1 part plant was macerated in 5 parts solvent). More concentrated tinctures (e.g., 1:2) require lower dosages than more dilute ones (e.g., 1:10).
2. **Plant Type**: Each plant has a specific safe therapeutic dosage. Some herbs, such as chamomile, are gentler and tolerated even at higher doses, while others, such as St. John's Wort, require more care.
3. **Method of Intake**: Tinctures are generally taken diluted in water, herbal tea, or juice to reduce the perception of alcoholic taste and promote absorption.

GENERAL DOSING GUIDELINES
To calculate the correct dosage, we use the concept of drops per administration. A basic formula consists of:
- **Standard tinctures** (1:5): 20-30 drops diluted in water, 2-3 times daily.
- **Concentrated tinctures** (1:2): 10-15 drops diluted in water, 2 times a day.
- **Light tinctures** (1:10): 30-50 drops diluted in water, 3 times a day.

PERSONALIZED DOSAGE CALCULATION
A precise approach is based on body weight, following the rule:
0.5 ml of tincture for every 10 kg of body weight.

For example:
- A 60 kg person takes about 3 ml of tincture per dose.
- An 80 kg person takes about 4 ml of tincture per dose.

CONVERSION OF MILLILITERS TO DROPS
For more convenient dosing, milliliters can be converted to drops. On average:
1 ml = 20 drops.

For example: 3 ml of tincture corresponds to 60 drops.

AGE- AND CONDITION-SPECIFIC DOSAGES
- **Healthy adults**: 20-30 drops per dose, 2-3 times daily.
- **Children (6-12 years)**: Reduce dosage to half, 10-15 drops per dose, diluted in water.
- **Elderly**: Start with 10-15 drops per dose, increasing gradually if necessary, under medical supervision.

EXAMPLE OF DOSAGE FOR DIFFERENT PLANTS
1. **Echinacea**: 20-30 drops every 2-3 hours at the first signs of a cold (up to 5 doses per day).
2. **Valerian**: 10-20 drops before bedtime to promote sleep.
3. **Calendula** (internal use): 10-15 drops 2 times daily to relieve internal inflammation.
4. **Hypericum**: 15-20 drops in the morning and at noon to support mood (avoiding evening dosage to avoid insomnia).

DOSAGE PRECAUTIONS.
1. **Overdose**: Taking tinctures in excessive doses can lead to unwanted side effects, such as stomach upset, nausea or hypotension.
2. **Duration of Treatment**: Most tinctures should not be used for periods longer than 8 consecutive weeks without

consulting a physician or herbalist.
3. **Allergies and Interactions**: Always check for personal allergies or drug interactions, especially for plants such as St. John's Wort or hawthorn.

USEFUL TOOLS FOR DOSING
1. **Dropper**: For accurately measuring drops.
2. **Teaspoons**: 1 teaspoon corresponds to about 5 ml (100 drops).
3. **Reference Tables**: Always consult a reliable dosage guide specific to each plant.

Accurate dosing not only ensures safe treatment, but also maximizes the therapeutic benefits of tinctures, making your home pharmacy a powerful tool for wellness.

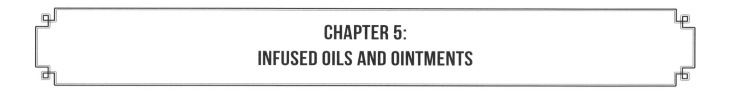

CHAPTER 5:
INFUSED OILS AND OINTMENTS

WHAT ARE INFUSED OILS AND OINTMENTS

Infused oils and ointments represent the beating heart of the home pharmacy. They are among the oldest and most versatile remedies, born from the combination of botanical wisdom and craftsmanship. These preparations combine the beneficial properties of plants with an oil or wax base, making them perfect for application to the skin and treatment of numerous ailments.

An infused oil is essentially an extract, obtained by soaking parts of plants-such as leaves, flowers, or roots-in a vegetable oil for a certain period of time. During this process, the plants' active substances, such as essential oils, flavonoids, and other bioactive molecules, transfer into the oil vehicle, creating a rich, therapeutic mixture. This extraction method is valued not only for its simplicity, but also for the gentleness with which it preserves the properties of the herbs, without the use of chemical solvents or high temperatures that could damage them. Infused oils can be used alone, directly on the skin, or as a base for creating other preparations, such as creams and ointments.

Ointments, on the other hand, are a more solid and stable form of preparation, made by mixing an infused oil with beeswax or another thickening agent. This makes them ideal for localized applications and skin protection, as they create a barrier that helps retain moisture and protect damaged areas. Ointments do not contain water, making them more durable than creams and lotions. Because of their waxy consistency, they can be applied without running, adhering to the skin for prolonged action. This characteristic makes them particularly useful for treating wounds, burns, cracked skin or muscle problems, as well as offering an excellent base for carrying active ingredients from specific plants.

On a practical level, infused oil and ointment are indispensable tools in the home pharmacy because of their ease of preparation and effectiveness. To create an infused oil, simply choose a quality vegetable oil-such as olive, almond, or jojoba oil-and combine it with a plant chosen according to the desired benefit. The oil, once the infusion process is complete, will have absorbed not only the therapeutic properties of the plant, but also its aroma and color. This characteristic makes infused oils a sensory delight as well as a healing remedy, evoking a deep connection with nature.

Ointments, with their fuller consistency, are often seen as "medicine in a jar." A simple calendula ointment, for example, can be a valuable ally in soothing skin irritations, while an arnica ointment can relieve muscle aches and bruises. The process of preparing ointments, although slightly more complex, is equally rewarding. It requires attention to temperature and a good deal of patience, as the dosage between oil and beeswax must be precisely calibrated to achieve the desired consistency.

The magic of these preparations lies in their ability to be customized. One infused oil or ointment is never the same: each jar tells a story, reflecting the personal choices of the herbalist, from the carefully gathered herbs to the base used. This flexibility allows anyone to create unique remedies, calibrated to their own or their family's needs. Moreover, the process of creating infused oils and ointments is not only a therapeutic art, but also a meditative act that promotes inner well-being. Preparing these blends with one's own hands is an experience that reconnects with the slow rhythm of nature, reminding us that healing and healing are not just a goal, but a path to be lived with awareness.

Infused oils and ointments thus offer a tangible and authentic approach to natural healing. Simple to prepare, effective and incredibly versatile, they are the foundation of a home pharmacy that aims for self-sufficiency and natural wellness.

Every drop of oil and every ounce of ointment encapsulates not only the benefits of plants, but also the loving intent of those who created them, transforming the remedy itself into an act of healing and connection.

INFUSED OILS FOR TOPICAL USE: SIMPLE RECIPES WITH LAVENDER, CALENDULA, AND ST. JOHN'S WORT

Infused oils for topical use are one of the most versatile and beloved preparations in the home pharmacy. They are gentle yet potent remedies, perfect for treating skin, relieving muscle aches or simply giving the gift of a relaxing moment. Using herbs such as lavender, calendula, and St. John's Wort, it is possible to create oils with soothing, anti-inflammatory, and restorative properties, suitable for a wide range of daily applications. Each infused oil is unique, as it encapsulates the specific properties of the chosen plant, transforming them into a ready-to-use solution.

LAVENDER: RELAXATION IN A BOTTLE

Lavender infused oil is known for its calming and rejuvenating properties. Lavender, with its distinctive floral scent, is a universal herb that lends itself to treating a variety of conditions. A lavender-infused oil can be used to soothe skin irritations, reduce redness, or promote muscle relaxation after a stressful day. To prepare it, you need to pick fresh or dried lavender flowers and soak them in a base oil, such as sweet almond or jojoba oil. The choice of base oil is crucial: it should be light and easily absorbed by the skin.

Once the flowers are soaked, the container should be left in a warm, sunny place for at least two weeks, shaking it gently every day to facilitate extraction. The resulting infused oil can be filtered and stored in a dark bottle to preserve its aroma and therapeutic properties.

CALENDULA: THE SKIN HEALER

Calendula is known as the herb par excellence for skin care. Its anti-inflammatory and healing properties make it ideal for treating wounds, burns, eczema or dry skin. Preparing a calendula infused oil is simple and rewarding. Fresh or dried calendula flowers are placed in a glass jar, covered completely with a nourishing vegetable oil, such as olive or sunflower seed oil.

This preparation is left to sit in a warm place, such as a sunny windowsill, for about three weeks. The natural heat speeds up the infusion process, allowing the beneficial compounds of calendula to transfer into the oil. After filtering, the infused oil can be used directly on the skin or as a base for ointments and salves. Its soothing and restorative effect makes it a must-have for anyone who wants to treat skin problems naturally.

ST. JOHN'S WORT: THE OIL OF THE SUN FOR MUSCLE PAIN AND DAMAGED SKIN

Hypericum infused oil, often called "St. John's oil," is famous for its distinctive ruby red color and therapeutic properties. It is a powerful remedy for muscle aches, bruises, and nerve inflammation because of its anti-inflammatory and analgesic abilities.

In addition, it is excellent for accelerating the healing of wounds and superficial burns. Preparation requires fresh flowers of St. John's Wort, preferably picked during the summer solstice, when the plant is at its most potent. The flowers are soaked in olive or sweet almond oil and left to steep in the sun for about 4 to 6 weeks. This process not only extracts the active compounds but also gives the oil its characteristic deep red color. Once filtered, St. John's Wort oil is ready for use, but should be stored away from light to keep its properties intact.

APPLICATIONS AND PRACTICAL TIPS

Lavender, calendula and St. John's Wort infused oils are simple to prepare but extraordinarily effective. They can be applied directly to the skin for massage, used as remedies for irritation, or used as basic ingredients for more complex ointments.

It is important to remember that the quality of the herbs and base oil greatly affects the final result. Always choose fresh, high-quality ingredients to ensure a safe and effective product. Also, store infused oils in dark containers in a cool, dry place to preserve their effectiveness for several months. Preparing these oils is an art that not only enriches your home pharmacy, but allows you to connect with nature and the power of plants.

DETAILED RECIPES FOR INFUSED OILS AND OINTMENTS

Infused oils, enriched with the properties of medicinal herbs, are a valuable tool for the natural treatment of numerous ailments. Each plant has a unique history, botanical characteristics and specific benefits. Below you will find detailed recipes, botanical information, therapeutic properties, dosages and precautions for use. Also included at the end of each recipe is the process for turning the infused oil into an ointment.

1. LAVENDER INFUSED OIL

Lavandula angustifolia
Family: Lamiaceae

Botanical characteristics: Lavender is an herbaceous perennial plant with small, intense purple flowers, gathered in spikes. It grows in temperate climates and is known for its calming aroma.

Therapeutic properties: Lavender is relaxing, soothing and antiseptic. Its oil is useful for relieving skin irritation, reducing inflammation and promoting muscle relaxation. It is ideal for treating small wounds, burns, and reducing stress.

RECIPE:
Ingredients:
- 30 g dried lavender flowers
- 200 ml base oil (sweet almond or jojoba)

Procedure:
1. Fill a glass jar with the lavender flowers, leaving at least 2 cm of space at the top.
2. Pour in the base oil until the flowers are completely covered. Stir gently to remove air bubbles.
3. Close the jar and let it steep in a sunny place for 2 to 3 weeks. Shake daily.
4. Strain the oil with gauze, removing any plant residue. Store the oil in a dark bottle.

Dosage and precautions:
- Apply a few drops directly to the skin or add 10 ml of infused oil to a neutral cream.
- Avoid application to deep or open wounds. Do not use if allergic to flowers of the Lamiaceae family.

Ointment:
- 100 ml of lavender infused oil
- 15 g beeswax
    - o   Melt the beeswax in a water bath.
    - o   Slowly add the infused oil, stirring constantly until smooth.
    - o   Pour into a sterilized jar and allow to cool.

2. CALENDULA INFUSED OIL

Calendula officinalis
Family: Asteraceae

Botanical characteristics: Calendula is an annual plant with distinctive orange or yellow flowers, known for its hardiness and ability to thrive in various types of soil.

Therapeutic properties: It has anti-inflammatory, healing and antiseptic properties. Calendula oil is especially effective for treating dry, chapped skin, eczema, dermatitis and mild sunburn.

RECIPE:
Ingredients:
- 40 g dried calendula flowers
- 250 ml of extra virgin olive oil

Procedure:
1. Place the calendula flowers in a glass jar and cover them completely with olive oil.
2. Leave the jar in a warm place (such as a windowsill) for 3-4 weeks.
3. Strain the oil with a gauze, removing the flowers. Transfer the oil to a dark container to preserve it.

Dosage and precautions:
- Apply a small amount directly to the skin twice a day.
- Avoid if you have allergies to Asteraceae. Do not use on open wounds without medical supervision.

Ointment:
- *100 ml of oil infused with calendula*
- *20 g beeswax*
    - o Melt the wax in a double boiler.
    - o Add the infused oil and stir until the mixture is uniform.
    - o Pour into a sterilized container and let cool.

3. HYPERICUM INFUSED OIL

Hypericum perforatum
Family: Hypericaceae

Botanical characteristics: Hypericum is an herbaceous perennial plant with bright yellow flowers. It is known as "St. John's wort" because it is traditionally harvested around the time of the summer solstice.

Therapeutic properties: St. John's Wort oil is anti-inflammatory, analgesic and regenerative. It is indicated for muscle pain, bruises, mild burns and mild neuralgia.

RECIPE:
Ingredients:
- 50 g fresh flowers of St. John's Wort
- 200 ml olive or sunflower seed oil

Procedure:
1. Place the fresh flowers in a glass jar and cover with the base oil.
2. Seal the jar and place it in a sunny place for 4-6 weeks. The oil will turn deep red.
3. Strain the oil with gauze and store it in a dark bottle.

Dosage and precautions:
- Apply to sore or inflamed areas once or twice a day.
- Avoid sun exposure after application, as St. John's Wort may increase sensitivity to light. Do not use during pregnancy.

Ointment:
- 100 ml of oil infused with St. John's Wort

- 20 g beeswax
  - o Melt the beeswax in a water bath.
  - o Add the infused oil and mix well.
  - o Pour the mixture into sterilized jars and let cool before use.

4. ARNICA INFUSED OIL

Arnica montana
Family: Asteraceae

Botanical characteristics: Arnica is an herbaceous perennial plant with yellow or orange, daisy-like flowers. It grows wild in mountainous, well-drained soils.

Therapeutic properties: Arnica oil is known for its anti-inflammatory and analgesic properties. It is useful for treating bruises, sprains, muscle pain and rheumatism.

RECIPE:
Ingredients:
- 30 g of dried arnica flowers
- 200 ml of base oil (sunflower or sweet almond oil)

Procedure:
1. Place the dried flowers in a glass jar and cover with the base oil.
2. Leave the infusion in a warm place for 2-3 weeks, gently shaking the jar daily. ·
3. Strain the oil with gauze and transfer it to a dark bottle for storage.

Dosage and precautions:
- Apply with gentle massage to skin in affected areas.
- Do not use on injured skin or open wounds. Avoid in case of allergy to Asteraceae.

Ointment:
- 100 ml of oil infused with arnica
- 15 g beeswax
  - o Melt the beeswax in a water bath.
  - o Add the infused oil, stirring until smooth.
  - o Pour into sterilized jars and let cool.

5. CHAMOMILE INFUSED OIL

Matricaria chamomilla
Family: Asteraceae

Botanical characteristics: Chamomile is an annual plant with small white flowers and a deep yellow center. It grows easily in meadows and well-drained soils.

Therapeutic properties: It has calming, soothing and anti-inflammatory properties. Chamomile oil is ideal for sensitive, irritated skin or skin prone to dermatitis. It is also effective for relieving muscle tension and cramps.

RECIPE:

Ingredients:
- 25 g of dried chamomile flowers
- 200 ml of base oil (jojoba or olive)

Procedure:
1. Place the chamomile flowers in a glass jar. Cover them completely with the base oil.
2. Place the jar in a warm place and let it sit for 2 weeks, shaking daily.
3. Strain the oil with gauze and transfer it to a dark container.

Dosage and precautions:
- Apply gently to the skin twice a day.
- Avoid use if you are allergic to plants in the Asteraceae family.

Ointment:
- 100 ml of oil infused with chamomile.
- 20 g beeswax
    - o Melt the wax in a double boiler and add the infused oil.
    - o Mix well and pour into sterilized jars.
    - o Let cool before sealing the jars.

6. PEPPERMINT INFUSED OIL

Peppermint
Family: Lamiaceae

Botanical characteristics: Peppermint is an herbaceous perennial plant with aromatic leaves and purplish flowers. It grows in moist, well-drained soils.

Therapeutic properties: Peppermint is refreshing, analgesic and antiseptic. The infused oil is useful for invigorating massages, relieving headaches and reducing muscle tension.

RECIPE:
Ingredients:
- 20 g fresh peppermint leaves
- 200 ml of base oil (grapeseed or olive oil)

Procedure:
1. Lightly crush the fresh peppermint leaves to release their essential oils.
2. Place the leaves in a glass jar and cover them with the base oil.
3. Let steep for 2 weeks in a cool, dark place.
4. Strain the oil with gauze and store in a dark bottle.

Dosage and precautions:
- Gently massage a small amount onto the temples to relieve headaches.
- Avoid contact with eyes and mucous membranes. Do not use on infants or young children.

Ointment:
- 100 ml peppermint infused oil.
- 15 g beeswax
    - o Melt the beeswax and add the infused oil.

o   Stir until the mixture is uniform.
o   Pour into sterilized jars and let cool.

7. THYME INFUSED OIL

Thymus vulgaris
Family: Lamiaceae

Botanical characteristics: Thyme is a small perennial shrub with aromatic leaves and white or pink flowers. It grows in dry, sunny soils.

Therapeutic properties: Thyme is antiseptic, antibacterial and anti-inflammatory. The infused oil is ideal for massages against colds and coughs, as well as for soothing muscle aches.

RECIPE:
Ingredients:
- 30 g fresh thyme leaves
- 250 ml of base oil (olive oil)

Procedure:
1. Place the thyme leaves in a glass jar and cover them completely with the base oil.
2. Leave the jar in a warm place for 3 weeks, shaking occasionally.
3. Strain the oil with gauze and transfer to a dark container.

Dosage and precautions:
- Massage on chest to relieve respiratory congestion.
- Avoid if you have allergies to Lamiaceae. Do not use during pregnancy without medical advice.

Ointment:
- 100 ml of oil infused with thyme
- 20 g beeswax.
    - o   Melt the wax in a double boiler and add the oil.
    - o   Stir and pour into sterilized jars.
    - o   Let cool before using.

8. ROSEMARY INFUSED OIL

Rosmarinus officinalis
Family: Lamiaceae

Botanical characteristics: Rosemary is an evergreen perennial shrub with needle-shaped leaves and blue-violet flowers. It grows in dry, sunny soils.

Therapeutic properties: Rosemary is invigorating, stimulating and analgesic. Rosemary infused oil is especially effective for improving circulation, relieving muscle aches and pains, and strengthening the scalp.

RECIPE:
Ingredients:
- 30 g fresh or dried rosemary leaves

- 200 ml of base oil (olive or grapeseed oil)

Procedure:
1. Lightly crush the rosemary leaves to release their essential oils.
2. Place the leaves in a glass jar and cover them completely with the base oil.
3. Place the jar in a warm place and let it steep for 3 weeks, shaking daily.
4. Strain the oil with gauze and transfer to a dark bottle.

Dosage and precautions:
- Apply a few drops to tired muscles or massage the scalp to stimulate hair growth.
- Avoid use on sensitive or irritated skin. Do not use during pregnancy or on children under 12 years of age.

Ointment:
- 100 ml of oil infused with rosemary
- 15 g beeswax
    o Melt the beeswax in a double boiler and add the infused oil.
    o Stir until evenly mixed and pour into sterilized jars.
    o Let cool before using.

9. SAGE INFUSED OIL

Salvia officinalis
Family: Lamiaceae

Botanical characteristics: Sage is an herbaceous perennial plant with gray-green leaves and blue or purple flowers. It is hardy and grows easily in sunny, well-drained soils.

Therapeutic properties: Sage is antiseptic, antifungal and invigorating. The infused oil is useful for treating skin infections, excessive sweating and muscle aches.

RECIPE:
Ingredients:
- 25 g dried sage leaves
- 200 ml of base oil (olive oil or sweet almond oil)

Procedure:
1. Place the sage leaves in a glass jar and cover with the base oil.
2. Place the jar in a warm place for 2 weeks, shaking gently every day.
3. Strain the oil and store it in a dark bottle to protect it from light.

Dosage and precautions:
- Apply a small amount to affected areas, maximum twice a day.
- Do not use during pregnancy or lactation. Do not apply to open wounds or severe burns.

Ointment:
- 100 ml of sage infused oil
- 20 g beeswax
    o Melt the wax in a double boiler, add the oil and mix well.
    o Pour into sterilized containers and let cool.

10. NETTLE INFUSED OIL

Urtica dioica
Family: Urticaceae

Botanical characteristics: Nettle is a perennial plant with serrated leaves and urticating hairs. It grows wild in nitrogen-rich soils.

Therapeutic properties: Nettle infused oil is rich in minerals and has anti-inflammatory and revitalizing properties. It is useful for stimulating circulation, relieving joint pain and strengthening hair.

RECIPE:
Ingredients:
- 30 g dried nettle leaves
- 200 ml of base oil (olive or coconut oil)

Procedure:
1. Place the nettle leaves in a glass jar and cover them completely with the oil.
2. Let it steep in a cool, dark place for 3 weeks.
3. Strain the oil and store it in a dark bottle.

Dosage and precautions:
- Massage into the scalp once a week or apply to sore joints.
- Avoid if you have sensitive skin or allergies.

Ointment:
- 100 ml of nettle-infused oil.
- 20 g beeswax
    - o Melt the beeswax in a double boiler and add the oil, stirring thoroughly.
    - o Pour into sterilized jars and let cool.

11. HYPERICUM AND CALENDULA INFUSED OIL (BLEND FOR DAMAGED SKIN).

Characteristics: Combining St. John's Wort and calendula amplifies the healing and anti-inflammatory properties. This blend is ideal for treating cuts, grazes and irritated skin.

RECIPE:
Ingredients:
- 15 g fresh St. John's Wort flowers
- 15 g of dried calendula flowers
- 200 ml of base oil (olive oil)

Procedure:
1. Combine the hypericum and calendula flowers in a glass jar.
2. Cover with the base oil and let it steep in a sunny place for 4 weeks.
3. Strain the oil and store it in a dark bottle.

Dosage and precautions:
Apply a small amount to damaged or cracked skin. Avoid during pregnancy or on severe burns.

Ointment:
- 100 ml of infused oil (blend)
- 15 g beeswax

Follow the standard procedure for ointment, mixing wax and oil well.

12. GINGER INFUSED OIL

Zingiber officinale
Family: Zingiberaceae

Botanical characteristics: Ginger is a rhizomatous root native to tropical regions. It occurs as a gnarled rhizome, rich in essential oils and active substances.

Therapeutic properties: Ginger is warming, anti-inflammatory and stimulating. The infused oil is ideal for relieving muscle aches, improving circulation and combating tension caused by cold weather.

RECIPE:
Ingredients:
- 50 g fresh ginger root, washed and grated
- 200 ml of base oil (sesame or olive oil)

Procedure:
1. Place the grated ginger in a glass jar and cover it completely with the base oil.
2. Place the jar in a warm place, or heat the jar in a bain-marie over low heat for 2 hours (maximum 40-50°C).
3. Strain the oil with gauze and store in a dark bottle.

Dosage and precautions:
- Massage a small amount on sore muscles or joints.
- Avoid use on sensitive or irritated skin. Do not use during pregnancy without medical advice.

Ointment:
- 100 ml ginger-infused oil.
- 20 g beeswax.
  - o Melt the wax in a double boiler, add the oil and stir until evenly mixed.
  - o Pour into sterilized jars and let cool.

13. TURMERIC INFUSED OIL

Curcuma longa
Family: Zingiberaceae

Botanical characteristics: Turmeric is a deep yellow-orange colored rhizomatous root native to South Asia. It is rich in curcumin, a powerful natural anti-inflammatory.

Therapeutic properties: Turmeric is anti-inflammatory, antioxidant and healing. The infused oil is useful for relieving joint pain, reducing swelling and promoting healing of small cuts.

RECIPE:
Ingredients:

- 40 g fresh turmeric root, washed and thinly sliced
- 250 ml of base oil (coconut or olive oil)

Procedure:
1. Place the turmeric slices in a glass jar and cover them completely with the base oil.
2. Heat the jar in a bain-marie for 2 hours, maintaining a constant temperature of 50°C.
3. Strain the oil and transfer it to a dark container for storage.

Dosage and precautions:
- Apply to inflamed joints or areas.
- Turmeric can stain skin and tissues. Do not use if you have an allergy to Zingiberaceae.

Ointment:
- 100 ml turmeric-infused oil.
- 20 g beeswax
    o Melt the beeswax and mix with the infused oil.
    o Pour into sterilized containers and allow to cool.

14. DANDELION INFUSED OIL

Taraxacum officinale
Family: Asteraceae

Botanical characteristics: Dandelion is an herbaceous perennial plant with toothed leaves and bright yellow flowers that produce characteristic dandelions. It grows wild in meadows and fallow land.

Therapeutic properties: Dandelion is detoxifying, anti-inflammatory and soothing. The infused oil is useful for draining massages and relieving joint pain.

RECIPE:
Ingredients:
- 30 g fresh dandelion flowers
- 200 ml base oil (sunflower or olive oil)

Procedure:
1. Gather the fresh dandelion flowers and let them dry for a few hours to remove excess moisture.
2. Place the flowers in a glass jar and cover them completely with the base oil.
3. Let it steep in a warm place for 3 weeks.
4. Strain the oil and transfer it to a dark bottle.

Dosage and precautions:
- Massage a small amount on painful areas.
- Avoid use on injured skin or open wounds.

Ointment:
- 100 ml dandelion infused oil.
- 20 g beeswax.
    o Melt the wax in a double boiler and add the oil.

Stir and pour into sterilized jars.

15. YARROW INFUSED OIL

Achillea millefolium
Family: Asteraceae

Botanical characteristics: Yarrow is an herbaceous perennial plant with jagged leaves and small, white or pink flowers. It grows wild in meadows and fields.

Therapeutic properties: Yarrow is healing, anti-inflammatory and antiseptic. The infused oil is useful for treating small wounds, excoriations and irritated skin.

RECIPE:
Ingredients:
- 30 g fresh yarrow flowers
- 200 ml of base oil (sweet almond or olive oil)

Procedure:
1. Place yarrow flowers in a glass jar and cover completely with the base oil.
2. Let it steep in a sunny place for 4 weeks, shaking daily.
3. Strain the oil and store it in a dark container.

Dosage and precautions:
- Apply a small amount directly to the skin.
- Avoid use on very sensitive skin or skin allergic to Asteraceae.

Ointment:
- 100 ml of oil infused with yarrow
- 20 g beeswax
  - o   Melt the beeswax in a double boiler and add the oil.
  - o   Stir well and pour into sterilized jars.

16. GARLIC INFUSED OIL

Allium sativum
Family: Amaryllidaceae

Botanical characteristics: Garlic is a bulbous perennial plant with a pungent aroma, known for its many medicinal applications. It grows in well-drained, sunny soils.

Therapeutic Properties: Antibacterial, antifungal and antiviral, garlic infused oil is ideal for treating skin infections, improving circulation and relieving joint pain.

RECIPE:
Ingredients:
- 5-6 cloves of fresh garlic
- 200 ml of base oil (olive or sunflower oil)

Procedure:
1. Peel and lightly crush the garlic cloves to release their active ingredients.
2. Put the garlic in a glass jar and cover it completely with the base oil.

3. Heat the jar in a bain-marie for 2 hours over very low heat (do not exceed 50°C).
4. Strain the oil and store it in a dark bottle.

Dosage and precautions:
- Apply locally to infected or sore areas.
- Do not use on sensitive skin or open wounds. Avoid sun exposure after application.

Ointment:
- 100 ml of oil infused with garlic
- 15 g beeswax.
  - o Melt the wax in a double boiler, add the oil and mix well.
  - o Pour into sterilized jars and let cool.

17. GINSENG INFUSED OIL

Panax ginseng
Family: Araliaceae

Botanical characteristics: Ginseng is a fleshy root known for its adaptogenic and stimulating properties. It grows in cool, shady soils.

Therapeutic properties: Invigorating, energizing and anti-inflammatory, ginseng infused oil is useful for invigorating massages and relieving muscle fatigue.

RECIPE:
Ingredients:
- 30 g dried ginseng root, cut into pieces
- 200 ml base oil (jojoba or sweet almond oil)

Procedure:
1. Place the root pieces in a glass jar and cover with the base oil.
2. Let it steep in a warm place for 4 weeks, shaking daily.
3. Strain the oil and store it in a dark bottle.

Dosage and precautions:
- Apply to tired muscles or areas of tension.
- Do not use on sensitive skin. Consult a physician before use during pregnancy.

Ointment:
- 100 ml ginseng infused oil.
- 20 g beeswax.
  - o Melt the wax and add the infused oil.
  - o Mix well and pour into sterilized containers.

18. MILK THISTLE INFUSED OIL

Silybum marianum
Family: Asteraceae

Botanical characteristics: Milk thistle is a herbaceous plant with purple flowers and thorny leaves, typical of uncultivated, sunny soils.

Therapeutic properties: A depurative and antioxidant, milk thistle infused oil is useful for improving skin health and soothing irritation.

RECIPE:
Ingredients:
- 30 g ground milk thistle seeds
- 200 ml of base oil (olive oil)

Procedure:
1. Grind the milk thistle seeds to release their active ingredients.
2. Place them in a glass jar and cover with the oil.
3. Let it steep for 4 weeks in a warm place.
4. Strain the oil with gauze and store it in a dark container.

Dosage and precautions:
- Apply to dry or cracked skin.
- Avoid in case of allergy to Asteraceae.

Ointment:
- 100 ml of oil infused with milk thistle.
- 20 g beeswax.
  - o Melt the wax and mix with the infused oil.
  - o Pour into sterilized jars.

19. EUCALYPTUS INFUSED OIL

Eucalyptus globulus
Family: Myrtaceae

Botanical characteristics: Eucalyptus is an evergreen tree native to Australia with long, aromatic leaves.

Therapeutic properties: Antiseptic, decongestant and refreshing, eucalyptus infused oil is ideal for chest massages during colds and sinusitis.

RECIPE:
Ingredients:
- 20 g dried eucalyptus leaves
- 200 ml of base oil (olive or sunflower oil)

Procedure:
1. Place the leaves in a jar and cover with the oil.
2. Let it steep in a warm place for 3 weeks.
3. Strain the oil and store it in a dark bottle.

Dosage and precautions:
- Apply to chest and back to help breathing.
- Do not use on infants or young children.

Ointment:
- 100 ml of oil infused with eucalyptus.
- 15 g beeswax.
  - o   Melt the wax and mix with the infused oil.
  - o   Pour into sterilized jars and let cool.

20. LICORICE INFUSED OIL

Glycyrrhiza glabra
Family: Fabaceae

Botanical characteristics: Licorice is an herbaceous plant with sweet, aromatic roots. It grows in deep, well-drained soils.

Therapeutic properties: Anti-inflammatory, soothing and antispasmodic, licorice infused oil is useful for soothing irritated skin and relieving muscle tension.

RECIPE:
Ingredients:
- 40 g dried and chopped licorice root
- 200 ml of base oil (sweet almond oil or jojoba oil)

Procedure:
1. Place the licorice root in a glass jar and cover it with the base oil.
2. Heat in a double boiler for 2 hours, maintaining a constant temperature.
3. Strain the oil and store it in a dark container.

Dosage and precautions:
- Apply locally to irritated or sore areas.
- Do not use in cases of hypertension or pregnancy.

Ointment:
- 100 ml licorice infused oil.
- 20 g beeswax.
  - o   Melt the wax and mix with the oil.
  - o   Pour into jars and let cool.

21. HYPERICUM AND CHAMOMILE INFUSED OIL (SOOTHING BLEND)

Hypericum perforatum and Matricaria chamomilla
Families: Hypericaceae and Asteraceae

Botanical characteristics: Hypericum, known as "St. John's Wort," is an herbaceous plant with yellow flowers. Chamomile, on the other hand, is an annual herb with white and yellow daisy-like flowers.

Therapeutic properties: This blend combines the soothing, healing and anti-inflammatory properties of St. John's Wort and chamomile. It is ideal for treating mild burns, skin irritations and minor cuts.

RECIPE:
Ingredients:
- 15 g fresh flowers of St. John's Wort
- 15 g of dried chamomile flowers
- 200 ml of base oil (olive oil or sweet almond oil)

Procedure:
1. Combine the flowers of St. John's Wort and chamomile in a glass jar.
2. Cover with the base oil and place the jar in a warm place for 4 weeks.
3. Strain the oil with gauze and store in a dark bottle.

Dosage and precautions:
- Apply to irritated or cracked skin twice a day.
- Avoid sun exposure after use because of the hypericum.

Ointment:
- 100 ml of infused oil (blend)
- 20 g beeswax
    - Melt the beeswax and add the infused oil.
    - Pour into sterilized jars and let cool.

22. BURDOCK INFUSED OIL

Arctium lappa
Family: Asteraceae

Botanical characteristics: Burdock is a biennial plant with large heart-shaped leaves and fleshy roots that grow in moist soil.

Therapeutic properties: Burdock has purifying, anti-inflammatory and sebum-regulating properties. The infused oil is useful for treating acne, dandruff and scalp irritation.

RECIPE:
Ingredients:
- 40 g fresh burdock root, washed and grated
- 200 ml of base oil (jojoba or grapeseed oil)

Procedure:
1. Place the grated root in a glass jar and cover it with the base oil.
2. Let it steep in a water bath for 2 hours, maintaining a constant temperature of about 40°C (104°F).
3. Strain the oil and store it in a dark container.

Dosage and precautions:
- Massage into the scalp once a week to stimulate hair growth.
- Avoid use on sensitive skin or skin allergic to Asteraceae.

Ointment:
- 100 ml of burdock infused oil.
- 20 g beeswax
    - Melt the wax and mix with the infused oil.
    - Pour into sterilized containers and let cool.

23. MALLOW INFUSED OIL

Malva sylvestris
Family: Malvaceae

Botanical characteristics: Mallow is an herbaceous perennial plant with rounded leaves and purple flowers. It grows in rich, well-drained soils.

Therapeutic properties: Mallow is emollient, soothing and anti-inflammatory. The infused oil is especially useful for treating dry, chapped skin and irritation.

RECIPE:
Ingredients:
- 30 g dried mallow flowers and leaves
- 200 ml of base oil (olive oil or sweet almond oil)

Procedure:
1. Place flowers and leaves in a jar and cover with the base oil.
2. Let it steep for 3 weeks in a warm place.
3. Strain the oil with gauze and store in a dark bottle.

Dosage and precautions:
- Apply to irritated or dry areas twice a day.
- Do not use if allergic to Malvaceae.

Ointment:
- 100 ml of oil infused with mallow
- 20 g beeswax.
    - o Melt the wax and mix with the oil.
    - o Pour into sterilized jars and let cool.

24. OIL INFUSED WITH THYME AND ROSEMARY (INVIGORATING BLEND)

Thymus vulgaris and Rosmarinus officinalis
Family: Lamiaceae

Botanical characteristics: Thyme and rosemary are aromatic perennials with small, fragrant leaves, widely grown in sunny soils.

Therapeutic properties: This blend is stimulating, antiseptic and invigorating. It is ideal for energizing massages and improving blood circulation.

RECIPE:
Ingredients:
- 20 g fresh thyme leaves
- 20 g fresh rosemary leaves
- 200 ml of base oil (grapeseed or olive oil)

Procedure:
1. Combine the leaves in a jar and cover them with the base oil.

2. Heat in a bain-marie for 2 hours, maintaining a constant temperature.
3. Strain the oil and store in a dark container.

Dosage and precautions:
- Apply to tired muscles for a revitalizing massage.
- Avoid during pregnancy or on young children.

Ointment:
- 100 ml of infused oil (blend)
- 15 g beeswax.
  - o   Melt the wax and mix with the oil.
  - o   Pour into sterilized jars and let cool.

25. CALENDULA AND LAVENDER INFUSED OIL (CALMING BLEND)

Calendula officinalis and Lavandula angustifolia
Family: Asteraceae and Lamiaceae

Botanical characteristics: Calendula and lavender are flowering herbs that thrive in sunny soils.

Therapeutic properties: This blend combines the calming and soothing properties of lavender with the healing and anti-inflammatory properties of calendula. It is ideal for sensitive and irritated skin.

RECIPE:
Ingredients:
- 20 g of dried marigold flowers
- 20 g of dried lavender flowers
- 200 ml of base oil (sweet almond oil)

Procedure:
1. Combine the flowers in a jar and cover with the base oil.
2. Let it steep in a sunny place for 3 weeks.
3. Strain the oil and store it in a dark bottle.

Dosage and precautions:
- Apply to irritated or reddened skin.
- Avoid use if you have allergies to the plants included.

Ointment:
- 100 ml of infused oil (blend)
- 20 g beeswax.
  - o   Melt the wax in a double boiler and mix with the infused oil.
  - o   Pour into sterilized containers and let cool.

BASIC OINTMENTS: A GUIDE FOR BURNS, WOUNDS AND MUSCLE PAIN

Ointments are solid, nourishing preparations that combine the beneficial properties of infused oils with the protection and effectiveness of beeswax. Due to their waxy consistency, ointments remain on the skin, creating a protective barrier that retains moisture and allows prolonged action of the active ingredients. Here you will find specific recipes for basic ointments, ideal for burns, wounds and muscle aches, with detailed instructions for each use.

1. OINTMENT FOR MILD SUNBURN

Indications: This ointment is designed to soothe mild sunburn, such as sunburn or caused by accidental contact with hot surfaces. It is moisturizing, soothing and promotes skin regeneration.

Main ingredients:
- Calendula infused oil: soothes irritation and promotes healing.
- St. John's Wort infused oil: regenerating and healing.
- Beeswax: creates a protective barrier on the skin.

Recipe:
- 50 ml of calendula infused oil
- 50 ml of infused oil of St. John's Wort
- 20 g beeswax
- 5 drops of lavender essential oil (optional, for additional soothing action)

Procedure:
1. Melt the beeswax in a double boiler over low heat.
2. Add the infused oils and stir gently until smooth.
3. Remove from heat and add lavender essential oil (if desired).
4. Pour the still-liquid mixture into sterilized jars and allow to cool completely before sealing the lids.

Directions for use: Gently apply a small amount to the affected area, 2-3 times a day.
Precautions: Do not use on severe burns or open wounds without medical supervision.

2. WOUND HEALING OINTMENT.

Indications: Ideal for minor cuts, scrapes and abrasions, this ointment speeds healing, protects against infection and soothes pain.

Main ingredients:
- Yarrow infused oil: healing and anti-inflammatory.
- Lavender infused oil: antiseptic and regenerating.
- Beeswax: protects the wound and maintains hydration.

Recipe:
- 50 ml of yarrow infused oil
- 50 ml of lavender infused oil
- 20 g beeswax
- 5 drops of tea tree essential oil (optional, for additional antibacterial action)

Procedure:
1. Melt the beeswax in a water bath, maintaining a constant, low temperature.

2. Add the infused oils and stir until evenly mixed.
3. Remove from heat and add tea tree essential oil (if using).
4. Pour ointment into sterilized jars and allow to cool completely.

Method of use: Apply a small amount directly to a clean, dry wound, 2 times a day.
Precautions: Do not use on deep or infected wounds without consulting a doctor.

3. WARMING OINTMENT FOR MUSCLE PAIN

Indications: This ointment is ideal for muscle aches and strains. With warming ingredients, it improves circulation and provides relief to sore muscles.

Main ingredients:
- Ginger infused oil: warming and anti-inflammatory.
- Rosemary infused oil: stimulating and decontracting.
- Beeswax: gives the ointment the right consistency.

Recipe:
- 50 ml of ginger infused oil
- 50 ml of oil infused with rosemary
- 20 g of beeswax
- 5 drops of eucalyptus essential oil (optional, for a cooling effect)

Procedure:
1. Melt the beeswax in a double boiler.
2. Add the infused oils and stir gently.
3. Remove from heat and, if desired, add eucalyptus essential oil.
4. Pour into sterilized jars and allow to cool.

Directions for use: Massage a small amount on the sore area 1-2 times a day.
Precautions: Avoid application on sensitive or irritated skin.

4. MULTIPURPOSE OINTMENT FOR IRRITATED SKIN.

Indications: A versatile treatment for redness, cracking and skin irritation.

Main ingredients:
- Calendula infused oil: anti-inflammatory and regenerating.
- Mallow infused oil: moisturizing and soothing.
- Beeswax: creates a protective barrier.

Recipe:
- 50 ml of calendula infused oil
- 50 ml of mallow infused oil
- 15 g beeswax

Procedure:
1. Melt the beeswax in a double boiler, add the oils and mix well.
2. Pour the mixture into sterilized jars and let cool.

Method of use: Apply a small amount to irritated or chapped areas, several times a day.
Precautions: Do not use on open wounds.

5. REFRESHING OINTMENT FOR BRUISES.

Indications: This ointment helps reduce swelling and bruising by providing a cooling and anti-inflammatory effect.

Main ingredients:
- Arnica infused oil: anti-inflammatory and soothing.
- Peppermint infused oil: cooling and analgesic.
- Beeswax: aids in localized application.

Recipe:
- 50 ml of arnica infused oil
- 50 ml peppermint infused oil
- 20 g of beeswax
- 5 drops of lavender essential oil (optional)

Procedure:
1. Melt the beeswax and add the infused oils, stirring until smooth.
2. Pour into sterilized jars and allow to cool.

Method of use: Apply gently to bruised areas 2 times a day.
Precautions: Avoid use on injured skin.

6. ANTIFUNGAL OINTMENT

Indications: This ointment is designed to treat fungal infections such as athlete's foot, mycoses, and other skin conditions caused by fungi.

Main ingredients:
- Tea tree infused oil: potent antifungal and antibacterial.
- Calendula infused oil: soothing and healing.
- Beeswax: seals the treated area and helps reduce moisture.

Recipe:
- 50 ml tea tree infused oil
- 50 ml of oil infused with calendula
- 20 g of beeswax
- 5 drops of eucalyptus essential oil (optional)

Procedure:
1. Melt the beeswax in a double boiler.
2. Add the infused oils and mix thoroughly.
3. If desired, add eucalyptus essential oil for additional action.
4. Pour into sterilized jars and allow to cool.

Directions for use: Apply a small amount to the affected area, 2-3 times a day.
Precautions: Do not use on injured skin or if allergic to essential oils.

7. OINTMENT FOR CHAPPED LIPS.

Indications: This moisturizing ointment is ideal for treating dry, chapped lips by creating a protective and nourishing barrier.

Main ingredients:
- Mallow infused oil: moisturizing and soothing.
- Shea butter: rich in fatty acids, nourishes and protects lips.
- Beeswax: helps maintain texture and creates a protective barrier.

Recipe:
- 50 ml of oil infused with mallow
- 30 g shea butter
- 15 g beeswax
- 5 drops of lavender or sweet orange essential oil (optional)

Procedure:
1. Melt the beeswax and shea butter in a double boiler.
2. Add the mallow-infused oil and stir until smooth.
3. Pour into small jars or lip sticks and let cool.

Directions for use: Apply to lips as often as needed.
Precautions: Do not use if allergic to ingredients.

8. SOOTHING OINTMENT FOR HEMORRHOIDS.

Indications: This ointment is designed to relieve the discomfort, irritation and swelling associated with hemorrhoids.

Main ingredients:
- St. John's Wort infused oil: regenerating and anti-inflammatory.
- Calendula infused oil: soothing and healing.
- Beeswax: provides texture and helps protect the skin.

Recipe:
- 50 ml hypericum infused oil
- 50 ml of calendula infused oil
- 20 g beeswax
- 5 drops of cypress essential oil (optional, to promote circulation)

Procedure:
1. Melt the beeswax in a double boiler.
2. Add the infused oils and mix well.
3. Pour into sterilized jars and let cool.

Method of use: Apply gently to the affected area 1-2 times a day.
Precautions: Consult a doctor in case of persistent symptoms.

9. ANTI-ITCH OINTMENT

Indications: Ideal for relieving itching caused by insect bites, skin allergies or dry skin.

Main ingredients:
- Lavender infused oil: soothing and regenerating.
- Peppermint infused oil: refreshing and soothing.
- Beeswax: protects and seals the treated area.

Recipe:
- 50 ml of lavender infused oil
- 50 ml peppermint infused oil
- 15 g beeswax
- 5 drops of blue chamomile essential oil (optional)

Procedure:
1. Melt the beeswax in a double boiler.
2. Add the infused oils and stir until evenly mixed.
3. Pour into sterilized containers and allow to cool.

Method of use: Apply a small amount to the affected area as needed.
Precautions: Do not use on open or deep wounds.

10. NAIL STRENGTHENING OINTMENT.

Indications: This ointment helps strengthen brittle nails and moisturize cuticles.

Main ingredients:
- Lemon infused oil: rich in vitamin C, promotes nail growth.
- Rosemary infused oil: stimulates circulation and strengthens nails.
- Cocoa butter: moisturizing and nourishing.

Recipe:
- 50 ml of lemon infused oil
- 30 ml of rosemary infused oil
- 20 g of cocoa butter
- 15 g beeswax

Procedure:
1. Melt the beeswax and cocoa butter in a double boiler.
2. Add the infused oils and mix thoroughly.
3. Pour into sterilized containers and allow to cool.

Directions for use: Massage a small amount on nails and cuticles each night before bedtime.
Precautions: Do not use if you have allergies to essential oils or ingredients.

11. DECONGESTANT OINTMENT FOR COLDS.

Indications: Perfect for relieving nasal congestion, coughs and chest tightness during colds and flu.

Main ingredients:
- Eucalyptus infused oil: decongestant and antiseptic.
- Peppermint infused oil: refreshing and soothing.
- Beeswax: gives texture and protects the skin.

Recipe:
- 50 ml of oil infused with eucalyptus
- 50 ml peppermint infused oil
- 20 g of beeswax
- 10 drops of camphor essential oil (optional)

Procedure:
1. Melt the beeswax in a double boiler.
2. Add the infused oils and essential oil, stirring well.
3. Pour into sterilized jars and allow to cool.

Directions for use: Massage a small amount on the chest and under the nose 2-3 times a day.
Precautions: Avoid use on children under 6 years of age and in cases of asthma.

12. JOINT PAIN RELIEF OINTMENT

Indications: Ideal for relieving joint pain, inflammation and stiffness.

Main ingredients:
- Arnica infused oil: anti-inflammatory and analgesic.
- Ginger infused oil: warming and relaxing.
- Beeswax: helps keep the compound on the skin.

Recipe:
- 50 ml of arnica infused oil
- 50 ml of ginger infused oil
- 20 g of beeswax
- 5 drops of rosemary essential oil (optional)

Procedure:
1. Melt the beeswax in a double boiler, add the infused oils and stir.
2. Pour into sterilized containers and allow to cool.

Method of use: Apply to aching joints, massaging gently.
Precautions: Do not use on irritated or injured skin.

13. OINTMENT FOR ECZEMA AND DERMATITIS.

Indications: A gentle treatment to soothe and moisturize skin affected by eczema or dermatitis.

Main ingredients:
- Chamomile infused oil: soothing and calming.
- Mallow infused oil: moisturizing and anti-inflammatory.
- Beeswax: creates a protective barrier on the skin.

Recipe:
- 50 ml of chamomile infused oil
- 50 ml of mallow infused oil
- 20 g of beeswax 5 drops of lavender essential oil (optional)

Procedure:
1. Melt the beeswax in a double boiler.
2. Add the infused oils and stir until a uniform consistency is achieved.
3. Pour into sterilized jars and allow to cool.

Directions for use: Apply gently to dry or irritated skin 1-2 times daily.
Precautions: Consult a doctor in case of severe eczema.

14. WARMING OINTMENT FOR COLD HANDS.

Indications: Perfect for those who suffer from cold hands due to cold weather or poor circulation.

Main ingredients:
- Ginger infused oil: warming.
- Rosemary infused oil: stimulating for circulation.
- Beeswax: maintains warmth on the skin.

Recipe:
- 50 ml of ginger infused oil
- 50 ml of rosemary infused oil
- 20 g beeswax

Procedure:
1. Melt the wax and add the infused oils, mixing well.
2. Pour into sterilized jars and let cool.

Method of use: Massage hands and fingers with a small amount of ointment.
Precautions: Do not use on irritated skin or with open wounds.

15. OINTMENT FOR INSECT BITES

Indications: Soothes itching and reduces swelling caused by insect bites.

Main ingredients:
- Lavender infused oil: soothing and calming.
- Peppermint infused oil: refreshing and antiseptic.
- Beeswax: helps seal the treated area.

Recipe:
- 50 ml of lavender infused oil
- 50 ml peppermint infused oil
- 15 g beeswax

Procedure:
1. Melt the wax and add the infused oils, mixing thoroughly.
2. Pour into sterilized jars and let cool.

Method of use: Apply directly to the sting 2-3 times a day.
Precautions: Do not use near the eyes.

16. SCAR OINTMENT.

Indications: Reduces the appearance of scars and improves skin elasticity.

Main ingredients:
- Rosehip infused oil: regenerating and antioxidant.
- Lavender infused oil: soothing and healing.
- Beeswax: protects and moisturizes.

Recipe:
- 50 ml of rosehip infused oil
- 50 ml of lavender infused oil
- 20 g beeswax

Procedure:
1. Melt the wax and combine the infused oils, mixing well.
2. Pour into sterilized containers and let cool.

Method of use: Apply twice daily to scars.
Precautions: Do not use on open wounds.

17. MOISTURIZING OINTMENT FOR CHAPPED HANDS.

Indications: A nourishing ointment for dry, chapped hands.

Main ingredients:
- Calendula infused oil: moisturizing and regenerating.
- Shea butter: deeply nourishes the skin.
- Beeswax: maintains moisture.

Recipe:
- 50 ml of calendula infused oil
- 30 g of shea butter
- 15 g of beeswax

Procedure:
1. Melt the wax and shea butter in a double boiler.
2. Add the infused oil and mix well.
3. Pour into sterilized containers and let cool.

18. SOOTHING OINTMENT FOR SUNBURNS.

Indications: Soothes reddened and irritated skin from sunburn.

Main ingredients:
- Aloe vera infused oil: cooling and regenerating.
- Lavender infused oil: soothing and moisturizing.
- Beeswax: protects and gives texture.

Recipe:
- 50 ml of aloe vera infused oil
- 50 ml of lavender infused oil
- 20 g of beeswax

Procedure:
1. Melt the wax and combine the infused oils.
2. Pour into sterilized containers and allow to cool.

19. OINTMENT FOR TIRED FEET

Indications: Relaxes and refreshes feet after a busy day.

Main ingredients:
- Peppermint infused oil: refreshing and stimulating.
- Eucalyptus infused oil: decongestant.
- Beeswax: maintains hydration.

Recipe:
- 50 ml peppermint infused oil.
- 50 ml of oil infused with eucalyptus
- 20 g beeswax

20. ANTI-AGING OINTMENT

Indications: Helps reduce signs of aging and keep skin supple.

Main ingredients:
- Rosehip infused oil: regenerating.
- Lavender infused oil: soothing.
- Beeswax: gives texture.

Recipe:
- 50 ml of rosehip infused oil
- 50 ml of lavender infused oil
- 20 g of beeswax

Method of use: Apply to clean skin every evening.

21. RHEUMATISM OINTMENT

Indications: This ointment helps reduce inflammation and joint pain associated with rheumatism.

Main ingredients:
- Devil's claw infused oil: anti-inflammatory and analgesic.
- Rosemary infused oil: stimulates circulation and relieves pain.
- Beeswax: keeps the compound on the skin.

Recipe:
- 50 ml devil's claw infused oil
- 50 ml of rosemary infused oil
- 20 g of beeswax
- 5 drops of camphor essential oil (optional)

Procedure:
1. Melt the beeswax in a double boiler.
2. Add the infused oils and stir until a uniform consistency is achieved.
3. Pour into sterilized jars and allow to cool.

Directions for use: Massage onto sore areas 1-2 times daily.
Precautions: Do not use on injured or irritated skin.

22. PROTECTIVE OINTMENT FOR WIND AND COLD

Indications: Perfect for protecting the skin during the winter months by creating a barrier against wind and cold.

Main ingredients:
- Calendula infused oil: moisturizing and regenerating.
- Shea butter: deeply nourishes the skin.
- Beeswax: creates a protective barrier.

Recipe:
- 50 ml of calendula infused oil
- 30 g of shea butter
- 20 g of beeswax

Procedure:
1. Melt the beeswax and shea butter in a double boiler.
2. Add the calendula-infused oil and mix well.
3. Pour into sterilized containers and allow to cool.

Directions for use: Apply to hands or face before going outdoors.
Precautions: Do not use on oily or acne-prone skin.

23. OINTMENT FOR BRUISES AND CONTUSIONS.

Indications: Reduces swelling and accelerates the reabsorption of bruises.

Main ingredients:
- Arnica infused oil: reduces swelling and relieves pain.
- St. John's Wort infused oil: regenerating and anti-inflammatory.
- Beeswax: seals the treated area.

Recipe:
- 50 ml of arnica infused oil
- 50 ml of infused oil of St. John's Wort
- 20 g of beeswax

Procedure:
1. Melt the beeswax in a double boiler and add the infused oils.
2. Stir well and pour into sterilized jars.
3. Let cool completely before sealing the jars.

Method of use: Apply directly to the bruise 2-3 times a day.
Precautions: Do not use on open wounds or cuts.

24. ANTI-INFLAMMATORY OINTMENT FOR TENDONITIS

Indications: Ideal for relieving inflammation and pain associated with tendonitis or overexertion.

Main ingredients:
- Ginger infused oil: warming and anti-inflammatory.
- Devil's claw infused oil: relieves pain and inflammation.
- Beeswax: helps keep the compound on the skin.

Recipe:
- 50 ml of ginger infused oil
- 50 ml devil's claw infused oil
- 20 g beeswax

Procedure:
1. Melt the wax in a double boiler, add the oils and mix well.
2. Pour into sterilized containers and let cool.

Method of use: Apply to inflamed areas 1-2 times a day.
Precautions: Do not use on sensitive or irritated skin.

25. OINTMENT AGAINST CRACKED FEET.

Indications: Perfect for softening and moisturizing cracked and dry heels.

Main ingredients:
- Mallow infused oil: moisturizing and soothing.
- Cocoa butter: deeply nourishes the skin.
- Beeswax: seals moisture into the skin.

Recipe:
- 50 ml of mallow infused oil
- 30 g of cocoa butter
- 20 g of beeswax
- 5 drops of tea tree essential oil (optional, for antimicrobial action)

Procedure:
1. Melt the beeswax and cocoa butter in a double boiler.
2. Add the infused oil and stir until a uniform consistency is achieved.
3. Pour into sterilized jars and allow to cool.

Directions for use: Apply to clean, dry feet every evening, covering with cotton socks for best effect.
Precautions: Do not use on open wounds or severe infections.

PRACTICAL TIPS FOR PREPARING AND USING OINTMENTS

The preparation of ointments is an art that requires attention to detail and respect for the natural properties of the ingredients. For maximum benefit, always use high-quality infused oils and fresh, organic ingredients. Sterilize jars and utensils thoroughly to avoid contamination and ensure that your ointments are safe and long-lasting. Store finished products in dark containers in a cool, dry place to preserve their properties. Remember to always test a small amount of product on a limited area of the skin before applying it more extensively to rule out any allergic reactions. Finally, keep in mind that natural ointments are complementary: for more serious conditions, always consult a doctor or qualified professional.

CHAPTER 6:
HERBAL TEAS AND INFUSIONS - ANCIENT AND MODERN REMEDIES

Herbal teas and infusions are among the oldest and most valued natural remedies, rooted in the traditions of many cultures. These easy-to-prepare beverages encapsulate the power of plants in an accessible and gentle form, offering benefits ranging from physical health support to mental relaxation. Each cup of herbal tea tells a story of herbal knowledge passed down through time, which today is intertwined with the demands of modern life.

An herbal tea or infusion is made by extracting the properties of plants through soaking in hot water. The process, while simple, requires care: the infusion time, the temperature of the water and the amount of herbs used can significantly affect the result. Herbal teas are distinguished by their balanced combination of flavors and therapeutic properties. They often include herbs, flowers, roots or seeds that work synergistically to address specific health problems or to provide moments of pure pleasure and relaxation.

In ancient remedies, herbal teas were considered a sacred way to connect to nature and its healing power. In modern times, they have been rediscovered not only for their physical benefits, but also for their ability to encourage moments of mindfulness and calm in a busy life. From chamomile for evening relaxation to green tea for an energy boost, each plant has its own identity and role to play.

Today, through the fusion of tradition and innovation, we can customize herbal teas to meet unique needs. Preparation thus becomes a ritual that invites you to slow down and take care of yourself. Herbal teas and infusions continue to be a bridge between ancient plant wisdom and modern holistic wellness needs.

RELAXING HERBAL TEAS - CHAMOMILE, LINDEN, LEMON BALM, AND OTHER HERBS

Relaxing herbal teas have always been one of the most beloved remedies for relieving stress, calming the mind and promoting restful sleep. Each herb used in these preparations makes a unique contribution, creating blends that not only pamper the senses, but work deeply to restore emotional and physical balance. Their action is based on natural compounds that interact with the nervous system, slowing the body's rhythm and promoting a feeling of calm.

Chamomile is probably the best-known relaxing herb. Its small white and yellow flowers are rich in apigenin, a flavonoid that acts as a natural sedative, helping to reduce anxiety and promote quality sleep. Preparing chamomile herbal tea is a simple and intimate act, a ritual that invites relaxation. Simply soaking the flowers in hot water for a few minutes produces a delicate drink with a slightly sweet, floral flavor that is perfect before bedtime.

Lime, with its fragrant flowers, is another great ally for relaxation. Rich in mucilage and essential oils, it works not only by calming the mind, but also by soothing muscle tension and promoting respiratory well-being. A linden herbal tea is especially good in times of intense stress or when feeling a sense of physical and mental oppression.

Lemon balm, with its citrusy and refreshing aroma, is a plant that combines sweetness and effectiveness. Known for its calming action on the central nervous system, it is often used to reduce nervous tension, relieve stress headaches, and promote peaceful digestion. A cup of lemon balm can be a great ally for relaxing after a busy day.

Other relaxing herbs such as lavender, hawthorn, and passion flower further enrich the blends, each with unique properties. Lavender, for example, not only relaxes, but calms irritability and improves mood through its therapeutic aroma.

Hawthorn works on the heart, reducing nervous tachycardia and promoting a sense of inner peace, while passionflower is particularly good for insomnia related to anxiety states.

Creating a personalized relaxing herbal tea is an act that combines tradition and creativity. Different herbs can be combined to achieve a synergistic effect, dosing the flavors and aromas according to one's preferences. For example, a blend of chamomile, lemon balm, and lavender offers a calming and balanced action, while adding a pinch of linden intensifies the overall relaxing effect.

The key to getting the maximum benefit from relaxing herbal teas is the quality of the ingredients. Choose high-quality fresh or dried herbs, preferably organic, to ensure that they keep their active ingredients intact. Preparing a relaxing herbal tea is more than just a drink: it is a moment for yourself, an invitation to slow down, breathe deeply, and reconnect with your inner well-being.

5 BASIC RELAXING HERBAL TEA RECIPES

Relaxing herbal teas are simple to prepare and are a natural way to relieve stress and tension. Each recipe uses herbs known for their calming properties, promoting overall well-being and improving sleep quality.

1. CLASSIC CHAMOMILE HERBAL TEA

Ingredients:
- 2 teaspoons of dried chamomile flowers
- 250 ml hot water

Preparation: Bring the water to a boil, then let it cool slightly (about 90°C). Pour the water over the chamomile flowers in a cup or teapot. Cover and let steep for 5-7 minutes. Strain and enjoy slowly, preferably before bedtime.

Benefits: Reduces anxiety, promotes relaxation and improves sleep.

2. LIME AND LEMON BALM HERBAL TEA.

Ingredients:
- 1 teaspoon of linden blossoms
- 1 teaspoon of lemon balm leaves
- 250 ml hot water

Preparation: Heat the water until it reaches boiling point, then pour it over the herbs in a cup. Cover and let steep for 7-10 minutes. Strain and drink slowly, preferably at a relaxing time in the evening.
Benefits: Calms the nervous system, relieves tension and promotes peaceful digestion.

3. LAVENDER RELAXING HERBAL TEA

Ingredients:
- 1 teaspoon dried lavender flowers
- 1 teaspoon of chamomile flowers
- 250 ml hot water

Preparation: Bring water to a boil and pour over the herbs in a cup or teapot. Cover and let stand for 5 to 7 minutes. Strain and enjoy slowly, letting the soothing aroma of lavender envelop you.
Benefits: Reduces irritability, calms the mind and improves mood.

4. PASSIONFLOWER AND HAWTHORN HERBAL TEA.

Ingredients:
- 1 teaspoon of passion flower leaves and flowers
- 1 teaspoon hawthorn flowers
- 250 ml hot water

Preparation: Bring the water to a temperature near boiling and pour it over the herbs. Cover and let steep for 8-10 minutes. Strain and sip slowly, preferably before bedtime.
Benefits: Relieves anxiety, promotes deep sleep and regulates heart rate.

5. HONEY AND LEMON BALM HERBAL TEA.

Ingredients:
- 1 teaspoon lemon balm leaves
- 1 teaspoon of chamomile flowers
- 1 teaspoon honey (optional)
- 250 ml hot water

Preparation: Pour the hot water over the herbs and cover. Let steep for 5-7 minutes, then strain. Add honey to sweeten if desired and sip slowly.
Benefits: Relaxes the body, relieves stress headaches and promotes peaceful digestion.

RECIPES FOR RELAXING HERBAL TEAS WITH FLAVORFUL COMBINATIONS.

In addition to being relaxing, herbal teas can provide pleasant and enveloping taste experiences by combining soothing herbs with aromatic and flavorful ingredients. Here are five recipes that combine the pleasures of taste with the benefits of relaxing plants.

1. CHAMOMILE AND VANILLA HERBAL TEA.

Ingredients:
- 2 teaspoons dried chamomile flowers
- 1 vanilla pod (or 1 teaspoon of natural extract)
- 250 ml hot water

Preparation: Bring the water to a boil and pour over the chamomile flowers in a cup. Add the cut vanilla pod or natural extract. Cover and let steep for 7 to 10 minutes. Strain and enjoy a sweetly aromatic drink, perfect for the evening.
Benefits and Taste: Chamomile relaxes and calms, while vanilla adds a sweet, comforting touch.

2. LEMON BALM AND GINGER HERBAL TEA WITH HONEY.

Ingredients:
- 1 teaspoon dried lemon balm leaves
- 2-3 slices of fresh ginger
- 1 teaspoon honey (optional)
- 250 ml hot water

Preparation: Bring water to a boil and pour over the lemon balm leaves and ginger slices. Cover and let steep for 8-10 minutes. Strain and add honey for a sweet and spicy touch.

Benefits and Taste: Lemon balm calms the nervous system, while ginger adds a pleasant warmth and stimulates digestion.

3. LIME AND ORANGE HERBAL TEA.

Ingredients:
- 1 teaspoon dried linden blossoms.
- Peel of half an orange (untreated)
- 250 ml hot water

Preparation: Thinly slice the zest of the orange, avoiding the white part. Pour the hot water over the lime blossoms and zest in a cup. Cover and let steep for 10 minutes. Strain and enjoy.

Benefits and Taste: The linden relaxes and soothes, while the orange zest gives a lively citrus note.

4. LAVENDER AND LEMON HERBAL TEA

Ingredients:
- 1 teaspoon dried lavender flowers.
- 2 slices of lemon (untreated)
- 250 ml hot water

Preparation: Pour the hot water over the lavender flowers and lemon slices in a cup. Cover and let stand for 5-7 minutes. Strain and enjoy a delicate and fragrant herbal tea.

Benefits and Taste: Lavender calms nerves and reduces irritability, while lemon adds freshness and lightness.

5. PASSIONFLOWER AND COCOA HERBAL TEA.

Ingredients:
- 1 teaspoon of dried passion flower leaves and flowers
- 1 teaspoon ground cocoa beans or pure cocoa powder
- 250 ml hot water

Preparation: Combine the passion flower and cocoa beans in a cup and pour in the hot water. Cover and let steep for 8-10 minutes. Strain and enjoy this unique and enveloping herbal tea.

Benefits and Taste: Passionflower promotes relaxation and sleep, while cocoa adds a deep aroma and a touch of pleasure.

6. CHAMOMILE, APPLE AND CINNAMON HERBAL TEA.

Ingredients:
- 2 teaspoons dried chamomile flowers
- 2 slices of fresh (or dried) apple
- 1 cinnamon stick

Preparation: Bring water to a boil and pour over the ingredients in a teapot. Cover and let steep for 8-10 minutes. Strain and enjoy.
Benefits and Taste: Chamomile calms, apple adds sweetness and cinnamon gives a spicy, comforting touch.

7. LEMON BALM AND LAVENDER HERBAL TEA WITH VANILLA.

Ingredients:
- 1 teaspoon dried lemon balm leaves
- 1 teaspoon lavender flowers
- 1 teaspoon of natural vanilla extract

Preparation: Combine ingredients in a cup and pour hot water. Cover and let steep for 7 to 9 minutes. Strain and enjoy.
Benefits and Taste: Lemon balm and lavender calm the nervous system, while vanilla gives an enveloping sweetness.

8. LIME AND BERRIES HERBAL TEA.

Ingredients:
- 1 teaspoon of linden blossoms
- 1 teaspoon dried berries (blueberries, raspberries, currants)

Preparation: Pour hot water over the ingredients in a cup or teapot. Let steep for 8 to 10 minutes. Strain and sip.
Benefits and Taste: Lime relaxes and berries give a fruity, slightly tart note.

9. CHAMOMILE AND LEMON HERBAL TEA WITH GINGER.

Ingredients:
- 2 teaspoons of chamomile flowers
- 2 slices of fresh lemon
- 2 thin slices of fresh ginger

Preparation: Combine all ingredients in a cup, pour hot water and let steep for 8-10 minutes. Strain and enjoy hot or lukewarm.
Benefits and Taste: Chamomile calms, lemon refreshes and ginger warms, creating a balanced mix.

10. MINT, LIME AND HONEY HERBAL TEA.

Ingredients:
- 1 teaspoon dried mint leaves.
- 1 teaspoon of linden blossoms
- 1 teaspoon honey (optional)

Preparation: Pour hot water over herbs in a cup. Let steep for 7-9 minutes, then strain and add honey if desired.
Benefits and Taste: Mint refreshes and relaxes, linden calms, and honey sweetens.

11. LAVENDER AND PEACH HERBAL TEA

Ingredients:
- 1 teaspoon lavender flowers
- 2 slices of fresh or dried peach

Preparation: Combine ingredients in a cup, pour hot water and let stand for 8-10 minutes. Strain and enjoy.
Benefits and Taste: Lavender calms the mind, while peach gives sweetness and delicacy.

12. PASSIONFLOWER AND COCONUT HERBAL TEA.

Ingredients:
- 1 teaspoon of dried passion flower leaves and flowers
- 1 teaspoon dried coconut flakes

Preparation: Pour hot water over the ingredients in a cup, cover and let steep for 7 to 9 minutes. Strain and enjoy slowly.
Benefits and Taste: Passionflower promotes sleep, while coconut adds an exotic, sweet flavor.

13. CHAMOMILE AND COCOA HERBAL TEA.

Ingredients:
- 1 teaspoon of chamomile flowers
- 1 teaspoon ground cocoa beans or pure cocoa powder

Preparation: Mix ingredients in a cup, pour hot water and let steep for 7-8 minutes. Strain and savor.
Benefits and Taste: Chamomile relaxes, while cocoa adds depth and a touch of pleasure.

14. CUCUMBER MINT HERBAL TEA.

Ingredients:
- 1 teaspoon of mint leaves
- 2 slices of fresh cucumber

Preparation: Pour hot water over the ingredients in a cup or teapot, cover and let steep for 5-7 minutes. Strain and enjoy fresh or lukewarm.
Benefits and Taste: The mint refreshes and calms, while the cucumber adds a thirst-quenching, gentle note.

15. LEMON BALM, STRAWBERRY AND LEMON HERBAL TEA.

Ingredients:
- 1 teaspoon dried lemon balm leaves.
- 2 slices of fresh or dried strawberry
- 1 slice of lemon

Preparation: Combine ingredients in a cup, pour hot water and let stand for 7 to 9 minutes. Strain and sip.
Benefits and Taste: Lemon balm relaxes, strawberry adds sweetness and lemon adds a touch of freshness.

ENERGIZING INFUSIONS - GINGER AND LEMON, MINT AND LICORICE

Energizing infusions are a natural and healthy way to recharge the body and mind. Ideal for meeting the challenges of the day or countering moments of fatigue, these drinks combine herbs and ingredients that stimulate circulation, improve concentration and invigorate the body without the use of caffeine.

One of the most popular combinations is ginger and lemon. Ginger, with its spicy, warming flavor, is known for its ability to improve blood circulation, stimulate metabolism and fight fatigue. Lemon, rich in vitamin C and with a fresh taste, enhances the energizing effect of ginger, providing an infusion that awakens the senses and supports the immune system. Preparing this infusion is simple: just soak slices of fresh ginger and a slice of lemon in hot water for about 10 minutes. The result is a refreshing and vigorous drink, perfect for starting the day.

Another energizing infusion with an intriguing flavor is mint and licorice. Mint, with its fresh, stimulating aroma, helps improve concentration and combat mental fatigue. Licorice, with its sweet and slightly spicy taste, acts as a natural tonic, invigorating the body and supporting the adrenal glands, which are often fatigued by prolonged stress. This combination creates a balanced and revitalizing infusion, great for the afternoon or during work breaks.

Energizing infusions are not limited to these two combinations. Lemon balm and rosemary, for example, combine the calming properties of the former with the stimulating effect of the latter, offering a blend that improves alertness and reduces fatigue. Turmeric and orange are another popular choice: turmeric, with its anti-inflammatory and revitalizing effect, marries with the citrusy freshness of orange, creating a warming and stimulating infusion.

Preparing an energizing infusion is not only a way to benefit from the properties of plants, but also a moment of self-care. These drinks, full of natural flavors and properties, are a healthy and enjoyable alternative to commercial energizing drinks, supporting the body in a balanced way without side effects.

RECIPES FOR ENERGIZING INFUSIONS

Energizing infusions are a combination of herbs, spices and other natural ingredients that stimulate the body and mind. These infusions are perfect to start the day, tackle a busy afternoon, or recharge naturally.

1. GINGER AND LEMON INFUSION

Ingredients:
- 3-4 slices of fresh ginger
- 1 slice of organic lemon
- 250 ml hot water

Preparation: Bring water to a boil and pour over the ginger and lemon in a cup. Let steep for 8-10 minutes, strain and enjoy.
Benefits: Stimulates metabolism, improves circulation and gives instant energy.

2. MINT AND LICORICE INFUSION

Ingredients:
- 1 teaspoon fresh or dried mint leaves
- 1 teaspoon dried licorice root
- 250 ml hot water

Preparation: Pour the hot water over the ingredients in a cup, cover and let steep for 10 minutes. Strain and sip slowly.
Benefits: Refreshes the mind and invigorates the body, promoting concentration.

3. TURMERIC AND ORANGE INFUSION

Ingredients:
- 1 teaspoon turmeric powder
- Peel of half an organic orange
- 250 ml hot water

Preparation: Combine turmeric and orange zest in a cup, pour in hot water and let stand for 7-8 minutes. Stir, strain and enjoy.
Benefits: Reduces inflammation and gives natural energy due to the freshness of the orange.

4. ROSEMARY AND LEMON INFUSION.

Ingredients:
- 1 teaspoon fresh rosemary leaves
- 1 slice of lemon
- 250 ml hot water

Preparation: Pour the hot water over the rosemary and lemon, cover and let steep for 10 minutes. Strain and enjoy.
Benefits: Stimulates circulation and improves concentration.

5. CINNAMON AND HONEY INFUSION.

Ingredients:
- 1 cinnamon stick or 1 teaspoon cinnamon powder
- 1 teaspoon honey (optional)
- 250 ml hot water

Preparation: Add cinnamon to hot water and let steep for 8-10 minutes. Strain, sweeten with honey and enjoy.
Benefits: Improves circulation and provides a gentle boost of natural energy.

6. GREEN TEA AND MINT INFUSION.

Ingredients:
- 1 teaspoon green tea leaves
- 1 teaspoon of mint leaves
- 250 ml hot water

Preparation: Pour hot (not boiling) water over green tea and mint. Let steep for 3-5 minutes, strain and enjoy.
Benefits: Increases energy and mental clarity due to the theine in green tea and the freshness of mint.

7. GINGER, CINNAMON AND CLOVE INFUSION.

Ingredients:
- 3 slices of fresh ginger
- 1 cinnamon stick
- 2 cloves
- 250 ml hot water

Preparation: Combine the ingredients in a cup and pour over the hot water. Cover and let steep for 10-12 minutes. Strain and enjoy.
Benefits: Warms and invigorates, improving circulation and physical energy.

8. POMEGRANATE AND GINGER INFUSION.

Ingredients:
- 2 tablespoons fresh pomegranate seeds
- 2 slices of fresh ginger
- 250 ml hot water

Preparation: Lightly crush the pomegranate seeds to release their juice and combine them with the ginger. Pour in the hot water, cover and let steep for 10 minutes. Strain and enjoy.
Benefits: Energizing and antioxidant, it helps fight physical and mental fatigue.

9. APPLE, LEMON AND CINNAMON INFUSION.

Ingredients:
- 2 slices of fresh apple
- 1 slice of lemon
- 1 cinnamon stick

Preparation: Combine the ingredients in a cup and pour over hot water. Cover and let steep for 10 minutes. Strain and enjoy.
Benefits: Invigorates and relaxes at the same time, offering a warm, enveloping flavor.

10. LICORICE AND ORANGE INFUSION.

Ingredients:
- 1 teaspoon dried licorice root.
- Peel of half an organic orange
- 250 ml hot water

Preparation: Combine the licorice and orange peel in a cup, pour in the hot water and let steep for 10 minutes. Strain and enjoy.
Benefits: Invigorating and sweetly spiced, it helps restore energy in times of fatigue.

MORE COMPLEX ENERGIZING INFUSIONS RECIPES

These recipes combine more sophisticated ingredients and sophisticated combinations to create energizing infusions with unique properties and more complex flavors.

1. EASTERN SPICE INFUSION

Ingredients:
- 3 slices of fresh ginger
- 1 cinnamon stick
- 2 crushed cardamom pods
- 1 clove
- 1 teaspoon honey (optional)
- 250 ml hot water

Preparation: Combine the spices in a teapot, pour in hot water and let steep for 12-15 minutes. Strain, sweeten with honey and enjoy slowly.
Benefits: This mixture warms, stimulates circulation and provides lasting energy.

2. MATCHA TEA AND LEMON INFUSION.

Ingredients:
- 1 teaspoon matcha tea powder
- 1 slice of lemon
- 1 teaspoon agave syrup (optional)
- 250 ml hot water (not boiling, about 80°C)

Preparation: Sift the matcha tea into a cup and add a little hot water to dissolve it, stirring well with a whisk or teaspoon. Add the remaining hot water, lemon slice and agave syrup.
Benefits: Rich in antioxidants and theine, this infusion improves concentration and provides steady energy.

3. ALPINE HERB INFUSION

Ingredients:
- 1 teaspoon dried yarrow leaves
- 1 teaspoon rosemary
- 1 teaspoon thyme
- 250 ml hot water

Preparation: Combine the herbs in a teapot, pour in hot water and let steep for 10 minutes. Strain and sip.
Benefits: This invigorating blend helps fight physical and mental fatigue, thanks to the mix of stimulating herbs.

4. BLACK TEA, ORANGE AND SPICE INFUSION.

Ingredients:
- 1 teaspoon black tea (Darjeeling or Assam).
- Peel of half an organic orange
- 1 cinnamon stick

- 2 crushed cardamom pods
- 250 ml hot water

Preparation: Pour the hot water over the tea and spices, cover and let steep for 4-5 minutes. Strain and enjoy.
Benefits: Black tea stimulates the nervous system, while the combination of orange and spices adds warmth and energy.

5. TURMERIC, GINGER AND COCONUT MILK INFUSION.

Ingredients:
- 1 teaspoon turmeric powder
- 3 slices of fresh ginger
- 200 ml hot water
- 50 ml coconut milk
- 1 teaspoon honey (optional)

Preparation: Combine turmeric, ginger and water in a pot and heat over low heat for 10 minutes. Add coconut milk and honey, stir well and strain.
Benefits: Energizing and anti-inflammatory, this infusion is ideal for a morning boost.

6. LICORICE, MINT AND EUCALYPTUS INFUSION.

Ingredients:
- 1 teaspoon dried licorice root.
- 1 teaspoon of mint leaves
- 1 teaspoon of eucalyptus leaves
- 250 ml hot water

Preparation: Pour the hot water over the ingredients and let steep for 8-10 minutes. Strain and enjoy.
Benefits: Invigorating and refreshing, it helps clear the respiratory tract and gives energy.

7. CITRUS AND GINGER INFUSION WITH ROSEMARY.

Ingredients:
- Peel of half an orange and half a lemon
- 3 slices of fresh ginger
- 1 sprig of fresh rosemary
- 250 ml hot water

Preparation: Combine ingredients in a teapot, pour in hot water and let stand for 10 minutes. Strain and sip slowly.
Benefits: Energizing and rich in vitamin C, this infusion stimulates the mind and invigorates the body.

8. GUARANA, GREEN TEA AND BERRIES INFUSION.

Ingredients:
- 1 teaspoon guarana powder
- 1 teaspoon green tea leaves
- 1 teaspoon dried berries

- 250 ml hot water

Preparation: Pour hot water over the ingredients and let steep for 5-7 minutes. Strain and enjoy.
Benefits: Guarana is a powerful natural stimulant, while green tea and berries provide antioxidants.

9. WHITE TEA, VANILLA AND LAVENDER INFUSION.

Ingredients:
- 1 teaspoon white tea
- 1 vanilla pod (or 1 teaspoon natural extract)
- 1 teaspoon dried lavender flowers
- 250 ml hot water (80°C)

Preparation: Combine the ingredients in a teapot, pour in the hot water and let steep for 3-5 minutes. Strain and enjoy.
Benefits: Delicate and elegant, this infusion stimulates the senses and gives mental energy.

10. APPLE, CINNAMON AND GINGER INFUSION WITH TURMERIC.

Ingredients:
- 2 slices of dried apple
- 1 cinnamon stick
- 2 slices of fresh ginger
- 1 teaspoon turmeric powder
- 250 ml hot water

Preparation: Combine all ingredients in a teapot, pour in hot water and let steep for 12 to 15 minutes. Strain and enjoy hot or lukewarm.
Benefits: Warming and invigorating, it helps fight fatigue and improve mood.

11. COCOA, GINGER AND CHILI INFUSION.

Ingredients:
- 1 teaspoon ground cocoa beans or pure cocoa powder
- 2 slices of fresh ginger
- A pinch of chili powder
- 250 ml hot water

Preparation: Combine the cocoa, ginger and chili powder in a cup. Pour over the hot water and stir well. Let steep for 8-10 minutes, strain and enjoy.
Benefits: Cocoa stimulates mental energy, ginger improves circulation, and chili pepper adds a boost of vitality.

12. MATE, LEMON AND GINGER INFUSION.

Ingredients:
- 1 teaspoon of yerba mate leaves
- 2 slices of fresh ginger
- Peel of half an organic lemon
- 250 ml of hot water (80°C)

Preparation: Pour the hot water over the mate, ginger and lemon peel. Cover and let steep for 7-8 minutes. Strain and sip slowly.

Benefits: Mate is a natural source of caffeine, ideal for increasing physical and mental energy, while lemon and ginger add freshness and warmth.

13. GINSENG, HONEY AND MINT INFUSION.

Ingredients:
- 1 teaspoon dried ginseng root.
- 1 teaspoon of mint leaves
- 1 teaspoon honey
- 250 ml hot water

Preparation: Combine the ginseng and mint in a cup. Pour in the hot water and let steep for 10 minutes. Strain, add the honey and enjoy slowly.

Benefits: Ginseng is an adaptogen that improves stress resistance, while mint refreshes and stimulates concentration.

14. CINNAMON, VANILLA AND CLOVE INFUSION.

Ingredients:
- 1 cinnamon stick
- 1 vanilla pod or 1 teaspoon of natural extract
- 2 cloves
- 250 ml hot water

Preparation: Combine the ingredients in a teapot and pour in the hot water. Let steep for 12 to 15 minutes, strain and enjoy hot.

Benefits: This warm and aromatic mixture stimulates the senses, increases energy and gives a feeling of comfort.

15. ROOIBOS, TURMERIC AND GINGER INFUSION WITH ORANGE PEEL.

Ingredients:
- 1 teaspoon of rooibos
- 1 teaspoon turmeric powder
- 2 slices of fresh ginger
- Peel of half an organic orange
- 250 ml hot water

Preparation: Place the rooibos, turmeric, ginger and orange zest in a teapot. Pour in the hot water and let steep for 10-12 minutes. Strain and sip slowly.

Benefits: The caffeine-free rooibos offers natural antioxidants, while the turmeric and ginger stimulate metabolism and the orange adds a fresh, vitaminic note.

CUSTOM BLENDS - HOW TO CREATE BALANCED COMBINATIONS

Creating a custom blend of herbal teas and infusions is an art that combines knowledge of the properties of herbs with the pleasure of exploring unique flavors and aromas. A good blend is not just a collection of ingredients, but a harmonious balance that meets specific needs, both physical and emotional.

To begin creating a balanced combination, it is essential to be clear about the purpose of the herbal tea. Do you want to relax? Recharge your energy? Promote digestion? Each goal guides the choice of the main ingredients, which are the heart of the blend. For example, for a relaxing herbal tea, herbs such as chamomile, lemon balm and linden are good bases; for an energizing infusion, on the other hand, ginger, lemon and mint offer a good start.

After choosing the main ingredients, it is important to consider the complementary elements, which enrich the blend with secondary flavors and benefits. For example, in a relaxing herbal tea, adding a pinch of lavender or orange zest can create a pleasant aroma without altering the calming effect. In an energizing infusion, a touch of cinnamon or cloves can add depth and warmth to the drink.

Another crucial aspect is the balance of flavors. Each blend should contain at least three dimensions of flavor: a main note (such as the sweetness of chamomile or the spiciness of ginger), a supporting note (such as the coolness of mint or the floral of lavender), and a contrasting note (such as the slight bitterness of green tea or the acidity of lemon). This balance creates a complete sensory experience, making the herbal tea more palatable.

The proportion of ingredients is also critical. A good starting point is to use a ratio of 2:1 between the main and complementary ingredients. For example, for a relaxing blend, you could use two parts lemon balm and chamomile and one part lemon peel. It is also important to respect the specific infusion times for each ingredient, as some herbs release their active compounds faster than others.

Finally, do not forget to experiment and adapt the blends to your personal preferences. Each combination can be modified to intensify or mitigate certain characteristics, creating unique and tailored herbal teas. Customization is a creative process that is refined with time and experience.

Preparing a custom blend is not only a way to harness the therapeutic properties of herbs, but also an act of caring for oneself and others. Whether it is a relaxing herbal tea for the evening or an energizing infusion for the morning, each combination becomes a reflection of one's needs and creativity.

CHAPTER 7:
OINTMENTS, CREAMS, AND BALMS

PROTECTIVE BALMS FOR LIPS AND DRY SKIN

Protective balm is one of the easiest and most versatile remedies to prepare in your home pharmacy. Perfect for dealing with the rigors of winter or soothing chapped skin in any season, a good balm acts as a protective barrier, retaining moisture and repairing damage caused by external agents.

Natural balms have an advantage over commercial ones: they are free of synthetic additives and enriched with ingredients specifically chosen for their soothing and regenerative properties. Preparing them at home allows you to customize recipes to suit your needs, experimenting with nourishing oils, moisturizing butters and aromatic essential oils.

In this section, you will learn how to create a **protective balm for lips and dry skin**, perfect for dealing with cold, windy or dry air. Step-by-step recipes and tips on how to customize your balm to maximize its effectiveness will follow.

STEP-BY-STEP RECIPE: PROTECTIVE BALM FOR LIPS AND DRY SKIN

Ingredients (for about 6 jars of 10 ml):
- 15 g grated (or pelleted) beeswax
- 30 g of coconut oil
- 15 g shea butter
- 10 ml sweet almond oil (optional, for extra hydration)
- 5-10 drops of lavender essential oil (or another of your choice, such as peppermint or rose)

Tools Needed:
- A mortar and pestle (optional, for manually mixing small amounts)
- A small saucepan for the water bath
- A silicone spatula or spoon
- Clean, sterilized containers (e.g., glass or metal jars)
- A pipette or syringe to pour the liquid conditioner into the containers without waste.

Preparation:
1. **Prepare the tools and containers**
   o Sterilize the jars by boiling them in hot water for 10 minutes and drying them completely. This step is critical to avoid contamination of the conditioner.

2. **Melt the beeswax**
   o Place the beeswax in a small saucepan over a water bath. Heat over low heat, stirring gently with

> *Did you know?*
>
> *Beeswax was used by the ancient Egyptians to protect and heal the skin? This natural ingredient has stood the test of time because of its incredible protective properties.*

a silicone spatula, until the wax melts completely.

3. **Add the butters and oils**
   o Once the wax is completely liquid, add the coconut oil and shea butter. Gently stir until everything is melted and blended.
   o Add the sweet almond oil (if you are using it) and continue stirring.

4. **Remove from heat and add the essential oils.**
   o Remove the saucepan from the water bath. Let the mixture cool for about 1 minute to prevent excessive heat from degrading the essential oils.
   o Add the drops of lavender essential oil and mix well.

5. **Pour the balm into the containers.**
   o Using a pipette or syringe, pour the still-liquid balsam into the jars. Work quickly-the conditioner solidifies quickly as it cools.

6. **Let cool and seal**
   o Leave the jars open at room temperature for about 1 hour or until the balm has solidified completely.
   o Seal with lids and store in a cool, dry place.

Usage Tips:
- **For lips**: Apply a small amount with your fingertips whenever you feel dry or chapped lips.
- **For dry skin**: Use it on hands, elbows or other chapped areas, massaging gently.

Personalize Your Conditioner!
1. **For a cool, refreshing touch**: add peppermint essential oil (5 drops).
2. **For a soothing effect**: add chamomile or calendula essential oil.
3. **Natural color**: add a pinch of natural mica powder or beet juice for a lightly colored conditioner.

ADDITIONAL RECIPES FOR PROTECTIVE BALMS FOR LIPS AND DRY SKIN

1. SOOTHING CALENDULA BALM

Ingredients:
- 10 g beeswax
- 20 g of calendula-infused oil (you can infuse it yourself using calendula flowers and olive oil)
- 10 g of shea butter
- 5 drops of chamomile essential oil

Procedure:
1. Melt the beeswax in a double boiler.
2. Add the calendula-infused oil and shea butter. Stir until the mixture is smooth.
3. Remove from heat and add the chamomile essential oil.
4. Pour into sterilized containers and allow to cool.

Use: Great for soothing chapped skin, redness and irritation.

2. HONEY MOISTURIZING BALM.

Ingredients:
- 15 g beeswax

- 25 g sweet almond oil
- 10 g cocoa butter
- 1 teaspoon of organic honey

Procedure:
1. Melt the beeswax, almond oil and cocoa butter in a double boiler.
2. Remove from heat and incorporate honey, stirring vigorously to distribute evenly.
3. Pour the balm into jars and let cool.

Use: Perfect for particularly dry or chapped lips. The honey adds a natural moisturizing effect.

3. LAVENDER AND TEA TREE REGENERATING BALM.

Ingredients:
- 15 g beeswax
- 20 g coconut oil
- 10 g of mango butter
- 5 drops of lavender essential oil
- 3 drops of tea tree essential oil

Procedure:
1. Melt the beeswax, coconut oil and mango butter in a double boiler.
2. Add the essential oils when the mixture has cooled slightly.
3. Pour into containers and let cool.

Use: Ideal for lips or skin with minor chapped skin due to the regenerative properties of tea tree.

4. NOURISHING ROSE BALM.

Ingredients:
- 15 g beeswax
- 20 g of jojoba oil
- 10 g shea butter
- 5 drops of rose essential oil
- 1 pinch of rose colored mica (optional, for a touch of color)

Procedure:
  o   Melt the beeswax, jojoba oil and shea butter in a double boiler.

4. Add rose essential oil and, if desired, mica to color the balm.
5. Pour into jars and let cool.

Use: Perfect for those looking for an elegant, moisturizing balm with a delicate floral fragrance.

5. REFRESHING MINT BALM.

Ingredients:
- 10 g beeswax
- 15 g coconut oil

- 15 g castor oil (for a glossy effect)
- 5 drops of peppermint essential oil

Procedure:
1. Melt the beeswax, coconut oil and castor oil in a double boiler.
2. Add the peppermint essential oil.
3. Pour into containers and let cool.

Use: Ideal for dry lips during summer or for a cooling effect during the day.

TIPS FOR CUSTOMIZING
1. Replace shea butter with cocoa butter for a more nourishing effect.
2. Add a pinch of cinnamon powder for a balm that stimulates lip microcirculation.
3. Use citrusy essential oils (sweet orange, lemon) for a fresh scent, but only in small amounts to avoid sensitization.

MUSCLE RELIEF OINTMENTS

Muscle relief ointments are one of the most popular remedies in the home pharmacy, ideal for relieving muscle pain, stiffness and tension.

Made from natural ingredients such as arnica and devil's claw, these ointments take advantage of the plants' anti-inflammatory and soothing properties to act directly on sore areas.

These remedies are particularly useful after intense physical exertion, to relieve joint pain related to chronic conditions such as arthritis, or simply to massage fatigued muscles. Home preparation yields a product that is natural, without chemical additives, and easily customized to enhance its effectiveness.

In this section, we will explore how to prepare two main ointments: one based on arnica, ideal for bruises and muscle tension, and one based on devil's claw, known for its powerful anti-inflammatory effect. Both recipes will include variations and suggestions for adapting them to your needs.

KEY INGREDIENTS
1. Arnica montana: Renowned for relieving muscle pain, bruises and swelling.
2. Devil's claw (Harpagophytum procumbens): Ideal for joint pain and chronic inflammation.
3. Sweet almond or olive oil: As a base to carry the active ingredients of plants.
4. Beeswax: To create the creamy, protective consistency of the ointment.

Did you know?

Devil's claw has been used for centuries in traditional African medicines to relieve joint pain.

Its curious name comes from the shape of the hooks of its fruit.

STEP-BY-STEP RECIPE: ARNICA OINTMENT FOR MUSCLE RELIEF

Ingredients (for about 100 g of ointment):
- 20 g of grated beeswax
- 50 ml of arnica infused oil (you can prepare it by steeping dried arnica flowers in sweet almond or olive oil for 4-6 weeks)
- 20 ml of coconut oil
- 10 ml lavender or rosemary essential oil (optional)
- 5 drops of peppermint essential oil (for a cooling and soothing effect)

Tools Needed:
A small saucepan for the water bath
- A silicone spatula or spoon
- Sterilized glass containers (e.g., 50-mL jars)
- A pipette or syringe (optional, for precise pouring)

Preparation:
1. **Prepare the ingredients and containers**
   o Sterilize the jars by boiling them in hot water for 10 minutes. Let them dry completely.
   o Prepare all ingredients on hand: beeswax, arnica infused oil and essential oils.

2. **Melt the beeswax and oils.**
   o In a small saucepan over a water bath, melt the beeswax along with the coconut oil and arnica-infused oil. Stir gently with a spatula until smooth.

3. **Add the essential oils**
   o Remove the saucepan from the heat and let the mixture cool for 1-2 minutes.
   o Add the lavender or rosemary essential oil (optional) and peppermint essential oil. Stir well.

4. **Pour the ointment into the containers**
   o Pour the still-liquid mixture into the sterilized jars. Use a pipette or syringe to avoid waste.
   o Let cool at room temperature for 1-2 hours until the ointment solidifies completely.

5. **Seal and store**
   o Seal the jars with the lids and store in a cool, dry place. The ointment will last up to 6 months if stored properly.

Method of Use:
- Apply a small amount of ointment directly to the painful area.
- Massage gently until completely absorbed. Repeat 2-3 times daily.

Customize Your Ointment.
1. **For a more cooling effect**: add 2-3 drops of eucalyptus essential oil.
2. **For a warming effect**: replace peppermint with 5 drops of ginger or cinnamon essential oil.
3. **For sensitive skin**: use jojoba oil instead of coconut oil.

CUSTOMIZATIONS FOR ARNICA OINTMENT FOR MUSCLE RELIEF

1. ARNICA AND GINGER WARMING OINTMENT

Modify:
- Add 5 drops of ginger essential oil for a warming effect.

- Reduce peppermint oil to 3 drops to balance the freshness.
- Use sesame oil instead of coconut oil, as it is known for its warming properties.

Indicated for: Muscle pain caused by cold or joint stiffness.

2. SOOTHING ARNICA AND CHAMOMILE OINTMENT.

Modification:
- Replace the rosemary essential oil with 5 drops of Roman chamomile essential oil.
- Reduce the amount of beeswax to 15 g for a creamier consistency.
- Add 1 teaspoon aloe vera gel when the mixture has cooled slightly.

Indicated for: Muscle pain associated with mild inflammation and sensitive skin.

3. ANTI-INFLAMMATORY ARNICA AND TURMERIC OINTMENT.

Modify:
- Add ½ teaspoon turmeric powder to the mixture while melting the beeswax.
- Strain the mixture with fine gauze before pouring into jars to remove any remaining turmeric.
- Add 5 drops of frankincense essential oil to enhance the anti-inflammatory effect.

Indicated for: Joint pain and chronic inflammation.

4. ARNICA AND LAVENDER RELAXING OINTMENT.

Modify:
- Use lavender infused oil (made by steeping dried lavender flowers in sweet almond oil for 4-6 weeks) instead of coconut oil.
- Add 10 drops of lavender essential oil and 2 drops of vanilla essential oil for a calming scent.

Indicated for: Muscle pain from stress or accumulated tension.

5. ARNICA AND DEVIL'S CLAW OINTMENT COMBINATION.

Modification:
- Replace half of the arnica oil with devil's claw infused oil.
- Add 3 drops of wintergreen (gaultheria) essential oil for a natural analgesic effect.
- Reduce beeswax to 18 g and add 5 ml jojoba oil for a softer consistency.

Indicated for: Intense muscle pain and joint stiffness.

GENERAL TIPS
1. Color and texture: For a visual touch, add a pinch of golden mica for a shimmering ointment.
2. Extra Infused Herbs: Consider adding an infusion of St. John's Wort for nerve pain or calendula for soothing action.
3. Storage: Add 1-2 drops of vitamin E to extend the life of the ointment.

STEP-BY-STEP RECIPE: DEVIL'S CLAW OINTMENT FOR MUSCLE RELIEF

Ingredients (for about 100 g of ointment):
- 20 g grated beeswax
- 50 ml devil's claw infused oil (prepared by infusing dried devil's claw roots in sweet almond or olive oil for 4-6 weeks)
- 20 ml coconut oil
- 10 ml of wintergreen (gaultheria) essential oil
- 5 drops of ginger or rosemary essential oil (optional, for a warming effect)

Tools Needed:
- Water bath pot
- Silicone spatula or spoon
- Sterilized glass jars (e.g., 50 ml)
- Pipette or syringe (optional)

Preparation:
1. **Sterilize the containers**
   o Wash and sterilize jars by boiling in hot water for 10 minutes. Dry completely before use.

2. **Melt the beeswax and base oils.**
   o In a small saucepan over a water bath, melt the beeswax along with the coconut oil and devil's claw infused oil.
   o Stir gently with a silicone spatula until the mixture is even and lump-free.

3. **Add the essential oils**
   o Remove the saucepan from the heat and let it cool for 1-2 minutes.
   o Add wintergreen essential oil and, if desired, ginger or rosemary essential oil. Stir well to distribute the oils evenly.

4. **Pour into containers**
   o Quickly pour the liquid mixture into sterilized jars. Use a pipette or syringe for greater precision and to avoid waste.
   o Let cool at room temperature for at least 1 to 2 hours, until completely solidified.

5. **Seal and store**
   o Seal the jars with the lids and store the ointment in a cool, dry place. It has a shelf life of about 6 months if stored properly.

Method of Use:
- Apply a small amount of ointment to the affected area.
- Massage gently to promote absorption. Repeat 2-3 times daily.

Customization Tips.
1. **Soothing effect**: Add 3 drops of lavender essential oil for a relaxing aroma.
2. **Extra warming effect**: Increase drops of ginger essential oil to 10, but be careful for sensitive skin.
3. **For dry skin**: Add 10 ml shea butter for extra emollient action.

Safety Box:
1. Do not apply the ointment to open wounds or irritated skin.
2. Do a skin test before use, especially if using warming essential oils such as ginger or wintergreen.

CUSTOMIZED RECIPES FOR DEVIL'S CLAW OINTMENT FOR MUSCLE RELIEF

1. DEVIL'S CLAW AND TURMERIC ANTI-INFLAMMATORY OINTMENT

Modify:
- Add ½ teaspoon turmeric powder to the mixture while melting the beeswax and oils.
- Strain the mixture with gauze to remove any remaining turmeric.
- Replace the wintergreen essential oil with 5 drops of frankincense essential oil, known for its anti-inflammatory properties.

Indicated for: Chronic pain and joint inflammation.

2. DEVIL'S CLAW AND CAPSICUM WARMING OINTMENT.

Modify:
- Add 1 teaspoon of chili pepper (capsicum) infused oil to the mixture for an intense warming effect.
- Use 10 g of shea butter in place of 1 part coconut oil for a creamier consistency.
- Integrate 3 drops of cinnamon essential oil to enhance warmth and improve circulation.

Indicated for: Cold-related muscle pain or winter stiffness.

3. SOOTHING DEVIL'S CLAW AND CALENDULA OINTMENT.

Modify:
- Mix 30 ml of devil's claw infused oil with 20 ml of calendula infused oil for soothing action on muscles and skin.
- Replace wintergreen essential oil with 5 drops of Roman chamomile essential oil.
- Reduce the beeswax to 15 g for a lighter, easier to spread consistency.

Indicated for: Muscle pain associated with sensitive or reddened skin.

4. DEVIL'S CLAW AND LAVENDER RELAXING OINTMENT.

Modify:
- Replace coconut oil with 30 ml jojoba oil, ideal for delicate skin.
- Add 10 drops of lavender essential oil and 5 drops of rose essential oil for a relaxing scent.
- Supplement 1 teaspoon of vitamin E to increase the ointment's shelf life.

Suitable for: Evening massages to relax fatigued muscles and promote rest.

5. REFRESHING DEVIL'S CLAW AND MENTHOL OINTMENT.

Modify:
- Add 5 g of menthol crystals to the mixture while melting the beeswax and oils.
- Replace wintergreen essential oil with 5 drops of eucalyptus essential oil for a balsamic effect.
- Use grape seed oil instead of coconut oil for a lighter consistency.

Indicated for: Quick relief from muscle pain after strenuous physical activity.

PRACTICAL BOX: EXTRA TIPS
- Combined warming and cooling effect: Mix warming (ginger) and cooling (mint) essential oils.
- Natural color: Add a pinch of cocoa powder for a soft brown color and natural scent.
- Extended Preservation: Integrate 1-2 drops of grapefruit seed oil as a natural preservative.

SAFETY BOX:

Ointments with capsicum or menthol may cause sensation of intense heat or cold. Test on a small area of skin before use.

NOURISHING CREAMS — ALOE VERA AND COCONUT OIL

Nourishing creams made with aloe vera and coconut oil are an ideal solution for naturally moisturizing and regenerating the skin. Aloe vera is renowned for its soothing, moisturizing and regenerating properties, while coconut oil provides deep hydration and protective action against dryness.

This combination creates a light, non-greasy cream that absorbs easily, making it perfect for the face, hands and body. Ideal for all skin types, it is especially good for skin that is dry, irritated or in need of extra pampering.

In this section, we will explore how to make a nourishing cream with aloe vera and coconut oil, with customizable variations for different skin types.

BENEFITS OF INGREDIENTS
- Aloe vera: Rich in vitamins (A, C, E, B12) and minerals, it stimulates cell regeneration and calms irritation.
- Coconut oil: Moisturizing and antibacterial, it penetrates deep into the skin for an emollient effect.
Lavender essential oil (optional): Helps relax and soothe the skin.

STEP-BY-STEP RECIPE: NOURISHING CREAM WITH ALOE VERA AND COCONUT OIL

Ingredients (for about 150 ml of cream):
- 50 ml pure aloe vera gel (preferably fresh or organic)
- 30 ml coconut oil (preferably extra virgin and organic)
- 20 ml sweet almond oil (optional, for extra emollient action)
- 1 teaspoon of shea butter (optional, for extra nutrition)
- 5-10 drops of lavender or rose essential oil (optional, for a relaxing scent)
- ½ teaspoon liquid vitamin E (optional, as a natural preservative)

Tools Needed:
- A heat-resistant bowl
- Electric whisk or hand whisk
- Small saucepan for water bath
- Clean, sterilized container (preferably glass)

Preparation:

1. **Sterilize the container**
   - o Wash the small jar or container with hot soapy water, then sterilize it by boiling it for 10 minutes. Dry completely.

2. **Melt the coconut oil and shea butter.**
   - o In a water bath bowl, melt the coconut oil and shea butter over low heat, stirring gently with a spatula until smooth.

3. **Add the aloe vera gel.**
   - o Remove the bowl from the water bath and allow the mixture to cool slightly.
   - o Add the aloe vera gel a little at a time, stirring constantly with an electric mixer or hand whisk to emulsify the ingredients.

4. **Integrate the essential oils and vitamin E**
   - o Once the mixture has reached a creamy consistency, add the essential oil drops and vitamin E. Mix well to blend everything together.

5. **Pour the cream into the container**
   - o Transfer the nourishing cream into the sterilized container. Use a spatula to avoid waste and make sure everything is well distributed.

6. **Let cool and store**
   - o Let the container cool at room temperature for at least 1 hour. Seal with the lid and store in the refrigerator for up to 1 to 2 weeks if using fresh aloe vera gel.

Method of Use:

- Apply a small amount of cream to clean, dry skin.
- Massage gently until completely absorbed. Ideal for face, hands and body.

Nourishing Cream Customizations.

1. Oily skin: Replace coconut oil with jojoba oil for a lighter texture.
2. Sensitive skin: Add 3 drops of Roman chamomile essential oil for a soothing effect.
3. Extremely dry skin: Add 1 extra teaspoon of shea butter and replace sweet almond oil with avocado oil.
4. Refreshing effect: Add 2 drops of peppermint essential oil.

Safety:

1. If you use fresh aloe vera, be sure to remove the aloin (yellowish part present near the peel) well, which may cause irritation.
2. Test a small area of your skin before using essential oils, especially if you have sensitive skin.

VARIATIONS OF THE NOURISHING CREAM WITH ALOE VERA AND COCONUT OIL

1. REFRESHING MINT AND CUCUMBER CREAM.

Modifications:

- Replace 20 ml aloe vera gel with 20 ml fresh filtered cucumber juice.
- Add 3 drops of peppermint essential oil for a cooling effect.
- Reduce coconut oil to 20 ml and supplement 10 ml jojoba oil, ideal for combination or oily skin.

Suitable for: Moisturizing and refreshing the skin during summer.

2. ROSE AND SHEA BUTTER REGENERATING CREAM.

Modifications:
- Use 30 ml of aloe vera gel and 1 extra teaspoon of shea butter for a more nourishing effect.
- Add 5 drops of rose essential oil and 2 drops of geranium essential oil, both known to stimulate cell regeneration.
- Replace sweet almond oil with avocado oil for increased skin elasticity.

Suitable for: Dry and mature skin.

3. SOOTHING CHAMOMILE AND CALENDULA CREAM.

Modifications:
- Replace 20 ml of coconut oil with 20 ml of calendula-infused oil.
- Add 3 drops of Roman chamomile essential oil and 2 drops of lavender essential oil.
- Reduce the amount of shea butter to ½ teaspoon for a lighter consistency.

Suitable for: Sensitive, reddened or easily irritated skin.

4. LEMON AND GREEN TEA ILLUMINATING CREAM.

Modifications:
- Add 1 teaspoon of green tea infused oil (prepared by steeping green tea leaves in jojoba oil).
- Add 2 drops of lemon essential oil and 3 drops of sweet orange essential oil.
- Reduce the aloe vera gel to 40 ml for a thicker consistency.

Suitable for: Dull or stressed skin, for an illuminating effect.

5. PROTECTIVE CREAM WITH HONEY AND PROPOLIS

Modifications:
- Add 1 teaspoon of organic honey to the mixture while mixing in aloe vera gel.
- Integrate 3 drops of propolis extract for protective action against external aggressions.
- Replace the essential oil with 2 drops of tea tree essential oil for a purifying effect.

Suitable for: Dry, chapped skin with a protective action against weathering.

SUGGESTIONS FOR CUSTOM VARIANTS.
- **For a lighter cream**: Reduce the shea butter and use a more fluid oil, such as grapeseed oil.
- **For an anti-aging effect**: Add 2 drops of frankincense essential oil and replace some of the coconut oil with argan oil.
- **For a calming effect**: Supplement a teaspoon of chamomile or calendula gel.

SECTION 3: NATURAL REMEDIES FOR COMMON AILMENTS

CHAPTER 8:
COMMON AILMENTS - HERBAL REMEDIES HANDBOOK

Home pharmacy is based on the idea that nature provides everything we need to support our health. Over the centuries, medicinal herbs have been used to relieve a wide range of ailments, often with amazing results. In this chapter you will find a detailed handbook of more than 250 herbal remedies, organized by type of ailment, so that you can quickly choose the best solution for each need.

This section is designed to be a practical and searchable companion, suitable both for those who want to address everyday problems such as headaches or insomnia, and for those seeking a natural remedy for specific ailments such as difficult digestion or joint pain. Each remedy has been selected for its effectiveness and safety, with clear directions on preparation and dosage.

In addition, you'll find helpful boxes with quick remedies and tips for creating your own mini-pharmacy so you're always ready to take natural action. Before you start, remember that knowledge is your best ally: always be well informed about the use of herbs, and consult an expert if you have any doubts or special conditions.

Whether you are seeking relief for yourself or want to care for your loved ones, this section will be the beating heart of your Home Apothecary. Get ready to discover the power and versatility of medicinal plants!

COLD AND COUGH — NATURAL REMEDIES

1. MALLOW (MALVA SYLVESTRIS) HERBAL TEA.

Ingredients: 1 tablespoon dried mallow flowers, 250 ml water.
Preparation: Bring water to a boil, add mallow flowers and let steep for 10 minutes. Strain before drinking.
Benefits: Mallow has emollient and anti-inflammatory properties, useful for soothing throat irritation and calming a dry cough .
Usage tips: Drink 2-3 cups a day.

2. THYME (THYMUS VULGARIS) INFUSION.

Ingredients: 1 teaspoon thyme flowering tops, 200 ml boiling water.
Preparation: Pour boiling water over thyme and cover. Let steep for 10 minutes and strain.
Benefits: Thyme has powerful antiseptic and balsamic properties, relieving coughs and colds.
Usage tips: Use as an herbal tea 2 times a day or as a mouthwash for an irritated throat.

3. DECOCTION OF HYSSOP (HYSSOPUS OFFICINALIS).

Ingredients: 2 teaspoons of hyssop flowering tops, 300 ml water.
Preparation: Boil the summits in water for 10 minutes, then strain.
Benefits: Expectorant and soothing, ideal for oily coughs or those with phlegm .

Usage tips: Drink hot 2 times a day.

4. ELDERBERRY (SAMBUCUS NIGRA) SYRUP.

Ingredients: 1 cup fresh or dried elderflowers, 1 liter water, 500 g sugar, 1 lemon.
Preparation: Bring water to a boil, add flowers and let macerate for 24 hours. Strain, add sugar and lemon juice. Heat until sugar is dissolved and store in bottle.
Benefits: Powerful sudorific and anti-inflammatory, useful for lowering fever and relieving colds .
Usage tips: Take 1 tablespoon 3 times a day.

5. INHALATION OF MINT (MENTHA PIPERITA).

Ingredients: 4-5 drops of mint essential oil, 1 liter of boiling water.
Preparation: Pour the essential oil into a bowl of boiling water. Cover your head with a towel and inhale deeply for 5-10 minutes.
Benefits: Natural decongestant, relieves nasal congestion and eases breathing .
Usage tips: Repeat 2 times a day.

6. ALTEA ROOT (ALTHAEA OFFICINALIS) DECOCTION.

Ingredients: 2 tablespoons dried marshmallow root, 500 ml water.
Preparation: Boil the root in water for 15 minutes, then strain.
Benefits: Mucilages in the root soothe irritated throat and reduce dry cough .
Usage tips: Drink lukewarm 2-3 times a day.

7. CHAMOMILE (MATRICARIA CHAMOMILLA) INFUSION.

Ingredients: 1 tablespoon chamomile flowers, 250 ml water.
Preparation: Pour boiling water over the flowers, cover and let steep for 10 minutes. Strain before drinking.
Benefits: Natural throat soother and mild sedative to promote rest .
Usage tips: Drink one cup before bedtime.

8. PLANTAIN (PLANTAGO MAJOR) INFUSION.

Ingredients: 2 teaspoons dried plantain leaves, 200 ml boiling water.
Preparation: Infuse the leaves for 10 minutes in boiling water and strain.
Benefits: Soothing for inflammation of the respiratory tract, useful against persistent cough.
Usage tips: Drink 2-3 times a day.

9. EUCALYPTUS INFUSION (EUCALYPTUS GLOBULUS).

Ingredients: 2 teaspoons of eucalyptus leaves, 300 ml water.
Preparation: Bring water to a boil and add the leaves. Let steep for 10 minutes and strain.
Benefits: Expectorant for phlegm, helps clear the respiratory tract.
Usage tips: Drink hot 1-2 times a day.

10. MALLOW MALLOW DECOCTION (MALVA MOSCHATA).

Ingredients: 2 tablespoons fresh or dried mallow mallow flowers, 300 ml water.
Preparation: Boil the flowers in water for 10 minutes, then strain.
Benefits: Relieves irritative cough and soothes inflammation of the throat.
Usage tips: Drink hot up to 3 times a day.

11. ELDERFLOWER AND LIME TREE HERBAL TEA.

Ingredients: 1 teaspoon elder flowers, 1 teaspoon linden flowers, 250 ml water.
Preparation: Infuse the herbs in boiling water for 10 minutes, then strain.
Benefits: Sweating and soothing for fever and cough.
Usage tips: Drink 2-3 cups a day, preferably hot.

12. HONEY AND LEMON SYRUP.

Ingredients: 3 tablespoons honey, juice of one lemon.
Preparation: Mix honey and lemon juice well. Store in a glass jar.
Benefits: Soothes irritated throat and calms cough.
Usage tips: Take one teaspoon every 2 to 3 hours.

13. INHALATIONS WITH THYME ESSENTIAL OIL.

Ingredients: 4-5 drops of thyme essential oil, 1 liter of boiling water.
Preparation: Pour the essential oil into the boiling water and inhale the vapors for 10 minutes.
Benefits: Natural antiseptic, helps clear the respiratory tract.
Usage tips: Repeat 2 times a day.

14. STAR ANISE (ILLICIUM VERUM) INFUSION.

Ingredients: 3-4 star anise, 250 ml water.
Preparation: Bring water to a boil, add aniseeds and let simmer for 10 minutes. Strain.
Benefits: Expectorant and soothing for coughs.
Usage tips: Drink hot 1-2 times a day.

15. LICORICE (GLYCYRRHIZA GLABRA) DECOCTION.

Ingredients: 1 teaspoon dried licorice root, 300 ml water.
Preparation: Boil the root in water for 15 minutes, then strain.
Benefits: Soothing for coughs and anti-inflammatory for the respiratory tract.
Usage tips: Drink 2-3 times a day.

16. HELICHRYSUM (HELICHRYSUM ITALICUM) INFUSION.

Ingredients: 1 tablespoon of helichrysum flowers, 250 ml water.
Preparation: Infuse the flowers in boiling water for 10 minutes and strain.

Benefits: Relieves cough and decongests the respiratory tract.
Usage tips: Drink 2 times a day.

17. EUCALYPTUS HONEY.

Ingredients: 1 teaspoon honey, 1 drop eucalyptus essential oil.
Preparation: Mix the essential oil into the honey.
Benefits: Decongestant and soothing to the throat.
Usage tips: Take in the morning and before bedtime.

18. GARGLE WITH SALT AND WATER.

Ingredients: 1 teaspoon salt, 200 ml lukewarm water.
Preparation: Mix salt in water and use to gargle.
Benefits: Reduces throat inflammation and fights bacteria.
Usage tips: Gargle 3 times a day.

19. VAPORS WITH BAY LEAVES.

Ingredients: 5-6 bay leaves, 1 liter of boiling water.
Preparation: Boil the leaves in the water and breathe in the vapors.
Benefits: Natural expectorant and soothing for the respiratory tract.
Usage tips: Repeat 2 times a day.

20. BASIL AND HONEY HERBAL TEA.

Ingredients: 1 teaspoon dried basil leaves, 1 teaspoon honey, 250 ml water.
Preparation: Infuse leaves in boiling water for 10 minutes, strain and add honey.
Benefits: Relieves sore throat and soothes cough.
Usage tips: Drink 2 times a day.

21. THYME AND SAGE LOTIONS

Ingredients: 2 teaspoons thyme and sage, 200 ml water.
Preparation: Boil the herbs in water, strain and use as a lotion.
Benefits: Antibacterial and antiseptic for throat and bronchi.
Usage tips: Use 3 times a day.

22. SCOTS PINE (PINUS SYLVESTRIS) SYRUP.

Ingredients: 1 cup fresh pine shoots, 500 ml water, 250 g sugar.
Preparation: Boil sprouts in water for 30 minutes, strain and add sugar. Heat until melted and store in a glass bottle.
Benefits: Expectorant and soothing for coughs.
Usage tips: 1 teaspoon 3 times a day.

23. DECOCTION OF ROSEMARY LEAVES (ROSMARINUS OFFICINALIS).

Ingredients: 1 teaspoon rosemary leaves, 250 ml water.
Preparation: Bring water to a boil, add leaves and let simmer for 5 minutes. Strain.
Benefits: Antiseptic and stimulating for the respiratory tract.
Usage tips: Drink hot 2 times a day.

24. ROSEMARY AND ALMOND OIL LOTION.

Ingredients: 2 teaspoons sweet almond oil, 5 drops rosemary essential oil.
Preparation: Mix ingredients and massage into chest to encourage breathing.
Benefits: Invigorating and decongesting, stimulates circulation in the respiratory tract.
Usage tips: Apply 2 times a day, in the morning and before bedtime.

25. INFUSION OF CALENDULA FLOWERS (CALENDULA OFFICINALIS).

Ingredients: 1 teaspoon calendula flowers, 250 ml boiling water.
Preparation: Infuse the flowers in boiling water for 10 minutes and strain.
Benefits: Soothing for irritated throat and anti-inflammatory.
Usage tips: Drink 2 times a day.

26. VAPORS WITH LAVENDER ESSENTIAL OIL (LAVANDULA ANGUSTIFOLIA).

Ingredients: 5 drops of lavender essential oil, 1 liter of boiling water.
Preparation: Pour the oil into the boiling water and breathe in the vapors for 10 minutes.
Benefits: Calming and decongestant.
Usage tips: Repeat 2 times a day.

27. GARGLE WITH SAGE INFUSION (SALVIA OFFICINALIS).

Ingredients: 1 tablespoon sage leaves, 200 ml water.
Preparation: Prepare an infusion by leaving the leaves in boiling water for 10 minutes. Strain and use to gargle.
Benefits: Disinfectant and soothing for irritated throat.
Usage tips: Gargle 3 times a day.

28. LEMON BALM AND LIME TREE HERBAL TEA.

Ingredients: 1 teaspoon lemon balm leaves, 1 teaspoon linden blossoms, 250 ml water.
Preparation: Infuse the herbs in boiling water for 10 minutes and strain.
Benefits: Cough soothing and relaxing.
Usage tips: Drink before bedtime.

29. GINGER AND CINNAMON SYRUP.

Ingredients: 1 teaspoon ginger powder, 1 cinnamon stick, 500 ml water, 3 tablespoons honey.
Preparation: Boil ginger and cinnamon in water for 10 minutes, strain and add honey.

Benefits: Warming and soothing to the throat.
Usage tips: 1 tablespoon 3 times a day.

30. FENNEL AND CLOVE DECOCTION.

Ingredients: 1 teaspoon fennel seeds, 3 cloves, 300 ml water.
Preparation: Boil seeds and cloves in water for 10 minutes, then strain.
Benefits: Expectorant and soothing for inflammation of the respiratory tract.
Usage tips: Drink hot 1-2 times a day.

31. ORIGANUM VAPORS (ORIGANUM VULGARE).

Ingredients: 1 teaspoon dried oregano, 1 liter boiling water.
Preparation: Add oregano to boiling water and breathe in the vapors.
Benefits: Expectorant and soothing to the respiratory tract.
Usage tips: Repeat 2 times a day.

32. BURDOCK (ARCTIUM LAPPA) DECOCTION.

Ingredients: 1 teaspoon dried burdock root, 300 ml water.
Preparation: Boil the root for 15 minutes, then strain.
Benefits: Anti-inflammatory and depurative, useful for reducing respiratory congestion.
Usage tips: Take hot, once a day.

33. GROUND IVY (GLECHOMA HEDERACEA) HERBAL TEA.

Ingredients: 1 teaspoon dried leaves of ground ivy, 250 ml boiling water.
Preparation: Infuse the leaves in boiling water for 10 minutes, then strain.
Benefits: Natural expectorant, helps clear the respiratory tract.
Usage tips: Drink hot 2 times a day.

34. ONION AND HONEY SYRUP.

Ingredients: 1 medium onion, 3 tablespoons honey.
Preparation: Cut onion into thin slices, alternate layers of onion and honey in a jar, let stand for 24 hours. Strain the liquid formed.
Benefits: Antibacterial and soothing for coughs.
Usage tips: Take 1 teaspoon 2-3 times a day.

35. INFUSION OF ENULA CAMPANA (INULA HELENIUM).

Ingredients: 1 teaspoon dried enula campana root, 300 ml water.
Preparation: Infuse the root in boiling water for 15 minutes and strain.
Benefits: Powerful expectorant, useful against phlegm and an oily cough.
Usage tips: Drink hot 1 time a day.

36. MYRTLE AND ALMOND ESSENTIAL OIL LOTION.

Ingredients: 5 drops of myrtle essential oil, 2 tablespoons of almond oil.
Preparation: Mix and use to massage the chest.
Benefits: Soothing for congestion and balsamic.
Usage tips: Apply before bedtime.

37. MARJORAM (ORIGANUM MAJORANA) VAPORS.

Ingredients: 1 tablespoon of marjoram leaves, 1 liter of boiling water.
Preparation: Pour boiling water over the leaves and breathe in the vapors.
Benefits: Calms cough and clears the respiratory tract.
Usage tips: Repeat 2 times a day.

38. DECOCTION OF WILLOW BARK (SALIX ALBA).

Ingredients: 1 teaspoon willow bark, 300 ml water.
Preparation: Boil the bark for 15 minutes, then strain.
Benefits: Anti-inflammatory and soothing to the respiratory tract.
Usage tips: Drink warm 1 time a day.

39. FARFARA (TUSSILAGO FARFARA) INFUSION.

Ingredients: 1 teaspoon dried leaves, 250 ml water.
Preparation: Infuse in boiling water for 10 minutes and strain.
Benefits: Bechic and soothing for dry coughs.
Usage tips: Drink 2-3 times a day.

40. LEMON AND HONEY BALM LOTION.

Ingredients: 1 teaspoon honey, juice of half a lemon.
Preparation: Mix ingredients and apply to chest.
Benefits: Improves breathing and calms cough.
Usage tips: Use the lotion before bedtime.

DIGESTION AND NAUSEA — NATURAL REMEDIES

Here is a collection of natural remedies to improve digestion and relieve nausea. Each remedy is detailed with ingredients, preparation and benefits.

1. GINGER (ZINGIBER OFFICINALE) INFUSION.

Ingredients: 1 teaspoon grated fresh ginger root, 250 ml boiling water.
Preparation: Pour boiling water over ginger and let steep for 10 minutes. Strain.
Benefits: Ginger stimulates digestion, relieves nausea and reduces abdominal cramps.

Usage tips: Drink hot after meals or as needed.

2. PEPPERMINT (MENTHA PIPERITA) INFUSION.

Ingredients: 1 teaspoon dried peppermint leaves, 250 ml boiling water.
Preparation: Infuse the leaves in boiling water for 10 minutes and strain.
Benefits: Peppermint aids digestion and relieves nausea and abdominal bloating.
Usage tips: Drink 2 times a day.

3. FENNEL (FOENICULUM VULGARE) DECOCTION.

Ingredients: 1 teaspoon fennel seeds, 300 ml water.
Preparation: Bring water with fennel seeds to a boil and simmer for 10 minutes. Strain.
Benefits: Helps reduce bloating, eases digestion and relieves nausea.
Usage tips: Drink hot after meals.

4. CHAMOMILE (MATRICARIA CHAMOMILLA) HERBAL TEA.

Ingredients: 1 tablespoon dried chamomile flowers, 250 ml boiling water.
Preparation: Pour boiling water over the flowers, cover and let steep for 10 minutes. Strain.
Benefits: Soothes the stomach, reduces abdominal cramps and relieves nausea.
Usage tips: Drink hot, before or after meals.

5. LEMON BALM INFUSION (MELISSA OFFICINALIS).

Ingredients: 1 tablespoon dried lemon balm leaves, 250 ml boiling water.
Preparation: Infuse leaves in boiling water for 10 minutes and strain.
Benefits: Relaxing and digestive, reduces heaviness and relieves nausea.
Usage tips: Drink 2 times a day, preferably after meals.

6. LEMON AND HONEY SYRUP.

Ingredients: Juice of 1 lemon, 3 tablespoons honey.
Preparation: Mix lemon juice with honey until a smooth syrup is obtained.
Benefits: Stimulates digestion and relieves mild nausea.
Usage tips: Take one teaspoon before or after meals.

7. GREEN ANISE INFUSION (PIMPINELLA ANISUM).

Ingredients: 1 teaspoon green anise seeds, 250 ml boiling water.
Preparation: Infuse seeds in boiling water for 10 minutes and strain.
Benefits: Promotes digestion and relieves nausea and abdominal bloating.
Usage tips: Drink hot after meals.

8. LICORICE ROOT (GLYCYRRHIZA GLABRA) DECOCTION.

Ingredients: 1 teaspoon dried licorice root, 300 ml water.
Preparation: Bring water with licorice root to a boil and simmer for 10 minutes. Strain.
Benefits: Calms nausea and aids digestion.
Usage tips: Drink hot once a day.

9. BERGAMOT ESSENTIAL OIL LOTION.

Ingredients: 3 drops bergamot essential oil, 1 teaspoon sweet almond oil.
Preparation: Mix the oils and gently massage into the solar plexus.
Benefits: Relaxes the stomach and helps reduce nausea.
Usage tips: Apply 2-3 times a day.

10. CORIANDER (CORIANDRUM SATIVUM) INFUSION.

Ingredients: 1 teaspoon coriander seeds, 250 ml boiling water.
Preparation: Infuse seeds in boiling water for 10 minutes and strain.
Benefits: Promotes digestion and reduces nausea.
Usage tips: Drink hot after meals.

11. SAGE (SALVIA OFFICINALIS) INFUSION.

Ingredients: 1 teaspoon dried sage leaves, 250 ml boiling water.
Preparation: Pour boiling water over the leaves, cover and let steep for 10 minutes. Strain before drinking.
Benefits: Aids digestion, reduces abdominal cramps and relieves nausea.
Usage tips: Drink 1-2 times a day, preferably after meals.

12. OREGANO (ORIGANUM VULGARE) HERBAL TEA.

Ingredients: 1 teaspoon dried oregano leaves, 250 ml boiling water.
Preparation: Infuse oregano in boiling water for 10 minutes and strain.
Benefits: Stimulates digestion and relieves abdominal bloating.
Usage tips: Drink hot after main meals.

13. ARTICHOKE (CYNARA SCOLYMUS) DECOCTION.

Ingredients: 1 teaspoon dried artichoke leaves, 300 ml water.
Preparation: Boil the leaves in water for 10 minutes, then strain.
Benefits: Improves liver function and relieves heaviness in the stomach.
Usage tips: Drink hot 1 time a day.

14. LAUREL HERBAL TEA (LAURUS NOBILIS).

Ingredients: 2-3 bay leaves, 250 ml boiling water.
Preparation: Pour boiling water over the leaves, cover and let steep for 10 minutes. Strain.

Benefits: Promotes digestion, relieves bloating and reduces nausea.
Usage tips: Drink hot after meals.

15. YARROW YARROW (ACHILLEA MILLEFOLIUM) INFUSION.

Ingredients: 1 teaspoon dried flowering tops, 250 ml boiling water.
Preparation: Infuse in boiling water for 10 minutes and strain.
Benefits: Relieves digestive discomfort and reduces nausea.
Usage tips: Drink hot 1-2 times a day.

16. CLOVE AND HONEY SYRUP.

Ingredients: 5 cloves, 250 ml water, 2 tablespoons honey.
Preparation: Boil cloves in water for 10 minutes, strain and add honey.
Benefits: Relieves nausea and aids digestion.
Usage tips: Take one teaspoon as needed.

17. GINGER AND MINT ESSENTIAL OIL LOTION.

Ingredients: 2 drops ginger essential oil, 2 drops mint essential oil, 1 tablespoon carrier oil.
Preparation: Mix the oils and massage the abdomen in circular motions.
Benefits: Reduces cramping and nausea.
Usage tips: Apply 2-3 times a day.

18. INFUSION OF CUMIN SEEDS (CUMINUM CYMINUM).

Ingredients: 1 teaspoon cumin seeds, 250 ml boiling water.
Preparation: Infuse seeds in boiling water for 10 minutes and strain.
Benefits: Reduces bloating and improves digestion.
Usage tips: Drink hot after meals.

19. GENTIAN (GENTIANA LUTEA) HERBAL TEA.

Ingredients: 1 teaspoon dried gentian root, 250 ml boiling water.
Preparation: Infuse the root in boiling water for 10 minutes and strain.
Benefits: Stimulates appetite and aids digestion.
Usage tips: Drink hot 1 time a day, before main meals.

20. ANGELICA ROOT (ANGELICA ARCHANGELICA) DECOCTION.

Ingredients: 1 teaspoon dried angelica root, 300 ml water.
Preparation: Bring water to a boil with the root, simmer for 10 minutes and strain.
Benefits: Promotes digestion and relieves nausea.
Usage tips: Drink hot once a day.

21. DILL SEED INFUSION (ANETHUM GRAVEOLENS)

Ingredients: 1 teaspoon dill seeds, 250 ml boiling water.
Preparation: Infuse seeds in boiling water for 10 minutes and strain.
Benefits: Promotes digestion and relieves bloating and abdominal cramps.
Usage tips: Drink hot 1-2 times a day.

22. CARDAMOM (ELETTARIA CARDAMOMUM) HERBAL TEA.

Ingredients: 1 teaspoon crushed cardamom seeds, 250 ml boiling water.
Preparation: Infuse the seeds in boiling water for 10 minutes and strain.
Benefits: Relieves nausea and stimulates digestion.
Usage tips: Drink hot after meals.

23. DANDELION ROOT DECOCTION (TARAXACUM OFFICINALE).

Ingredients: 1 teaspoon dried dandelion root, 300 ml water.
Preparation: Boil the root in water for 15 minutes and strain.
Benefits: Supports liver function and aids digestion.
Usage tips: Drink hot once a day.

24. LEMON AND LAVENDER ESSENTIAL OIL LOTION.

Ingredients: 3 drops lemon essential oil, 2 drops lavender essential oil, 1 tablespoon carrier oil.
Preparation: Mix the oils and gently massage the solar plexus.
Benefits: Relaxes the stomach and reduces nausea.
Usage tips: Apply 2 times a day.

25. PAPAYA SEED INFUSION.

Ingredients: 1 teaspoon dried papaya seeds, 250 ml boiling water.
Preparation: Infuse seeds in boiling water for 10 minutes and strain.
Benefits: Improves digestion and relieves heaviness.
Usage tips: Drink hot after meals.

26. ROMAN CHAMOMILE (ANTHEMIS NOBILIS) FLOWER HERBAL TEA.

Ingredients: 1 teaspoon dried Roman chamomile flowers, 250 ml boiling water.
Preparation: Infuse the flowers in boiling water for 10 minutes and strain.
Benefits: Soothes the stomach and aids digestion.
Usage tips: Drink warm before bedtime.

27. DECOCTION OF TURMERIC ROOT (CURCUMA LONGA).

Ingredients: 1 teaspoon grated fresh turmeric root, 300 ml water.
Preparation: Bring turmeric to a boil in water for 10 minutes and strain.

Benefits: Natural anti-inflammatory, stimulates digestion and relieves nausea.
Usage tips: Drink once a day.

28. ROSEMARY AND SAGE INFUSION.

Ingredients: 1 teaspoon rosemary leaves, 1 teaspoon sage leaves, 250 ml boiling water.
Preparation: Infuse the leaves in boiling water for 10 minutes and strain.
Benefits: Stimulates digestion and reduces abdominal bloating.
Usage tips: Drink hot after meals.

29. ANISE AND GINGER SYRUP.

Ingredients: 1 teaspoon anise seed, 1 teaspoon grated ginger root, 300 ml water, 2 tablespoons honey.
Preparation: Boil anise and ginger in water for 10 minutes, strain and add honey.
Benefits: Soothes the stomach and aids digestion.
Usage tips: Take one tablespoon as needed.

30. BASIL AND ALMOND OIL LOTION.

Ingredients: 2 drops basil essential oil, 1 tablespoon sweet almond oil.
Preparation: Mix the oils and gently massage into the abdomen.
Benefits: Reduces cramping and promotes stomach relaxation.
Usage tips: Apply 2-3 times a day.

31. INFUSION OF BIRCH LEAVES (BETULA PENDULA)

Ingredients: 1 teaspoon dried birch leaves, 250 ml boiling water.
Preparation: Infuse the leaves in boiling water for 10 minutes and strain.
Benefits: Improves digestion and helps reduce water retention related to bloating.
Usage tips: Drink 1-2 times a day.

32. HAWTHORN FLOWER HERBAL TEA (CRATAEGUS MONOGYNA).

Ingredients: 1 teaspoon dried hawthorn flowers, 250 ml boiling water.
Preparation: Infuse the flowers in boiling water for 10 minutes and strain.
Benefits: Relaxes the digestive system and helps reduce cramps.
Usage tips: Drink hot once a day.

33. LOTION WITH BLACK PEPPER AND MINT ESSENTIAL OIL.

Ingredients: 2 drops black pepper essential oil, 3 drops mint essential oil, 1 tablespoon sweet almond oil.
Preparation: Mix the oils and gently massage the abdomen.
Benefits: Stimulates digestion and reduces feelings of nausea.
Usage tips: Apply before main meals.

34. FENUGREEK SEED DECOCTION (TRIGONELLA FOENUM-GRAECUM).

Ingredients: 1 teaspoon fenugreek seeds, 300 ml water.
Preparation: Boil seeds in water for 10 minutes, then strain.
Benefits: Promotes intestinal transit and relieves bloating.
Usage tips: Drink once a day.

35. INFUSION OF HOLY BASIL LEAVES (OCIMUM TENUIFLORUM).

Ingredients: 1 teaspoon holy basil leaves, 250 ml boiling water.
Preparation: Infuse leaves in boiling water for 10 minutes and strain.
Benefits: Supports digestion and relieves nausea.
Usage tips: Drink hot after meals.

36. CUMIN AND CORIANDER SEED SYRUP.

Ingredients: 1 teaspoon cumin seeds, 1 teaspoon coriander seeds, 300 ml water, 2 tablespoons honey.
Preparation: Boil seeds in water for 10 minutes, strain and add honey.
Benefits: Stimulates digestion and reduces abdominal bloating.
Usage tips: Take one tablespoon 2 times a day.

37. JUNIPER AND SWEET ALMOND LOTION.

Ingredients: 3 drops juniper essential oil, 1 tablespoon sweet almond oil.
Preparation: Mix the oils and massage into the solar plexus.
Benefits: Stimulates digestion and relieves abdominal cramps.
Usage tips: Apply once a day.

38. VERBENA ODOROSA LEAF HERBAL TEA (ALOYSIA CITRODORA).

Ingredients: 1 teaspoon dried verbena leaves, 250 ml boiling water.
Preparation: Infuse the leaves in boiling water for 10 minutes and strain.
Benefits: Promotes digestion and calms heaviness.
Usage tips: Drink hot after main meals.

39. INFUSION OF GALANGA ROOT (ALPINIA GALANGA).

Ingredients: 1 teaspoon grated galanga root, 250 ml boiling water.
Preparation: Infuse the root in boiling water for 10 minutes and strain.
Benefits: Stimulates digestion and reduces nausea.
Usage tips: Drink hot once a day.

40. NETTLE LEAF (URTICA DIOICA) DECOCTION.

Ingredients: 1 teaspoon dried nettle leaves, 300 ml water.
Preparation: Boil the leaves in water for 10 minutes, then strain.

Benefits: Promotes digestive function and reduces bloating.
Usage tips: Drink once a day.

HEADACHE — NATURAL REMEDIES

Here is a selection of natural remedies to relieve headaches, each with details on ingredients, preparation and benefits.

1. INFUSION OF LEMON BALM LEAVES (MELISSA OFFICINALIS).

Ingredients: 1 teaspoon dried lemon balm leaves, 250 ml boiling water.
Preparation: Pour boiling water over the leaves and let steep for 10 minutes. Strain.
Benefits: Calming and relaxing, ideal for stress headaches.
Usage tips: Drink hot 1-2 times a day.

2. LAVENDER (LAVANDULA ANGUSTIFOLIA) ESSENTIAL OIL LOTION.

Ingredients: 2 drops lavender essential oil, 1 teaspoon sweet almond oil.
Preparation: Mix the oils and gently massage the temples and nape of the neck.
Benefits: Soothing and relaxing, relieves tension headaches.
Usage tips: Apply as needed.

3. MINT (MENTHA PIPERITA) LEAF POULTICE.

Ingredients: 5-6 fresh mint leaves, 100 ml water.
Preparation: Crush the leaves, soak them in warm water and apply to the forehead.
Benefits: Decongestant and refreshing, useful for localized headaches.
Usage tips: Keep the compress on the forehead for 15 minutes.

4. INFUSION OF CHAMOMILE FLOWERS (MATRICARIA CHAMOMILLA).

Ingredients: 1 tablespoon dried chamomile flowers, 250 ml boiling water.
Preparation: Pour boiling water over the flowers, cover and let steep for 10 minutes. Strain.
Benefits: Relaxing for head and neck muscles, relieves pain.
Usage tips: Drink hot once a day.

5. ROSEMARY ESSENTIAL OIL LOTION (ROSMARINUS OFFICINALIS).

Ingredients: 2 drops rosemary essential oil, 1 teaspoon carrier oil (e.g., almond oil).
Preparation: Mix the oils and gently massage into the scalp.
Benefits: Stimulates blood circulation and relieves headaches.
Usage tips: Apply as needed.

6. LIME TREE HERBAL TEA (TILIA CORDATA).

Ingredients: 1 teaspoon linden flowers, 250 ml boiling water.
Preparation: Infuse the flowers in boiling water for 10 minutes and strain.
Benefits: Relaxes the nervous system, ideal for stress headaches or insomnia.
Usage tips: Drink hot before bedtime.

7. VAPORS WITH PEPPERMINT ESSENTIAL OIL.

Ingredients: 4-5 drops of peppermint essential oil, 1 liter of boiling water.
Preparation: Pour the essential oil into a bowl of boiling water and breathe in the vapors for 10 minutes.
Benefits: Natural decongestant, useful for headaches related to sinusitis.
Usage tips: Repeat 1-2 times a day.

8. PASSIONFLOWER (PASSIFLORA INCARNATA) INFUSION.

Ingredients: 1 teaspoon dried passion flower leaves, 250 ml boiling water.
Preparation: Infuse the leaves in boiling water for 10 minutes and strain.
Benefits: Reduces nervousness and helps soothe tension headaches.
Usage tips: Drink one cup as needed.

9. RAW POTATO WRAP.

Ingredients: 1 medium potato.
Preparation: Thinly slice the potato and apply the slices to the forehead, covering with a cloth.
Benefits: Natural soothing properties, helps reduce pain.
Usage tips: Keep the compress on for 20 minutes.

10. DECOCTION OF WILLOW BARK (SALIX ALBA).

Ingredients: 1 teaspoon willow bark, 300 ml water.
Preparation: Boil the bark in water for 15 minutes, then strain.
Benefits: Contains salicin, a natural analgesic useful for headaches.
Usage tips: Drink hot once a day.

11. GINGER AND LEMON INFUSION

Ingredients: 1 teaspoon fresh grated ginger root, 250 ml boiling water, juice of half a lemon.
Preparation: Pour boiling water over ginger, let steep for 10 minutes, add lemon juice and strain.
Benefits: Anti-inflammatory and relaxing, reduces tension headaches and associated nausea.
Usage tips: Drink hot as needed.

12. BASIL ESSENTIAL OIL LOTION.

Ingredients: 3 drops basil essential oil, 1 teaspoon carrier oil (e.g., almond oil).
Preparation: Mix the oils and gently massage the temples and nape of the neck.

Benefits: Promotes muscle relaxation and relieves tension pain.
Usage tips: Apply as needed.

13. CABBAGE LEAF POULTICE.

Ingredients: 2-3 fresh cabbage leaves.
Preparation: Lightly crush the leaves with a rolling pin to release the juice and apply to the forehead, securing with a bandage.
Benefits: Natural anti-inflammatory properties, useful for pulsating headaches.
Usage tips: Keep the compress on for 20-30 minutes.

14. LAVENDER AND LIME BLOSSOM HERBAL TEA.

Ingredients: 1 teaspoon lavender flowers, 1 teaspoon linden flowers, 250 ml boiling water.
Preparation: Infuse the flowers in boiling water for 10 minutes and strain.
Benefits: Relaxing and calming, ideal for stress headaches.
Usage tips: Drink warm before bedtime.

15. VERBENA ODOROSA LEAF INFUSION (ALOYSIA CITRODORA).

Ingredients: 1 teaspoon dried verbena leaves, 250 ml boiling water.
Preparation: Pour boiling water over the leaves and let steep for 10 minutes. Strain.
Benefits: Relieves headaches and promotes mental relaxation.
Usage tips: Drink hot as needed.

16. EUCALYPTUS AND LAVENDER ESSENTIAL OIL LOTION.

Ingredients: 2 drops eucalyptus essential oil, 2 drops lavender essential oil, 1 tablespoon carrier oil.
Preparation: Mix the oils and gently massage the forehead and temples.
Benefits: Decongestant and relaxing, useful for sinus headaches.
Usage tips: Apply as needed.

17. DECOCTION OF ANGELICA ROOT (ANGELICA ARCHANGELICA).

Ingredients: 1 teaspoon dried angelica root, 300 ml water.
Preparation: Boil the root in water for 10 minutes, then strain.
Benefits: Stimulates circulation and relieves headaches.
Usage tips: Drink hot once a day.

18. CHAMOMILE OIL AND SALT POULTICE.

Ingredients: 1 tablespoon chamomile oil, 2 teaspoons fine salt.
Preparation: Mix the salt with the oil and apply the mixture to a gauze. Place the gauze on the forehead or temples.
Benefits: Relaxes muscles and reduces tension.
Usage tips: Keep the compress on for 15-20 minutes.

19. ROSEMARY AND MINT VAPOR.

Ingredients: 1 teaspoon rosemary leaves, 1 teaspoon mint leaves, 1 liter boiling water.
Preparation: Pour boiling water over the herbs and breathe in the vapors for 10 minutes.
Benefits: Decongestant and stimulating, relieves fatigue headaches.
Usage tips: Repeat once a day.

20. YARROW YARROW AND CHAMOMILE HERBAL TEA.

Ingredients: 1 teaspoon yarrow flowering tops, 1 teaspoon chamomile flowers, 250 ml boiling water.
Preparation: Infuse the herbs in boiling water for 10 minutes and strain.
Benefits: Relaxing and anti-inflammatory, useful for inflammation-related headaches.
Usage tips: Drink hot once a day.

21. INFUSION OF SAGE LEAVES (SALVIA OFFICINALIS)

Ingredients: 1 teaspoon dried sage leaves, 250 ml boiling water.
Preparation: Infuse the leaves in boiling water for 10 minutes, then strain.
Benefits: Relaxes the nervous system and helps relieve tension headaches.
Usage tips: Drink hot as needed.

22. MARJORAM (ORIGANUM MAJORANA) ESSENTIAL OIL LOTION.

Ingredients: 3 drops of marjoram essential oil, 1 teaspoon of carrier oil.
Preparation: Mix the oils and gently massage the temples and nape of the neck.
Benefits: Relaxes muscles and reduces pain.
Usage tips: Apply as needed.

23. GREEN CLAY AND ROSEMARY WATER POULTICE.

Ingredients: 2 tablespoons green clay, rosemary infusion.
Preparation: Mix the clay with the infusion until you get a paste and apply it to the forehead.
Benefits: Reduces inflammation and relieves throbbing headaches.
Usage tips: Leave on for 20 minutes and rinse.

24. INFUSION OF BIRCH BARK (BETULA PENDULA).

Ingredients: 1 teaspoon dried bark, 300 ml boiling water.
Preparation: Infuse the bark in boiling water for 15 minutes and strain.
Benefits: Natural anti-inflammatory, relieves pain and improves circulation.
Usage tips: Drink hot once a day.

25. YLANG YLANG ESSENTIAL OIL LOTION.

Ingredients: 2 drops of ylang ylang essential oil, 1 teaspoon of carrier oil.
Preparation: Mix the oils and gently massage into the temples.

Benefits: Relaxes the mind and reduces tension headaches.
Usage tips: Apply before bedtime.

26. ELDERFLOWER (SAMBUCUS NIGRA) DECOCTION.

Ingredients: 1 teaspoon elderflowers, 300 ml water.
Preparation: Boil the flowers in water for 10 minutes, then strain.
Benefits: Relaxes muscles and relieves symptoms of sinus headaches.
Usage tips: Drink hot once a day.

27. BAY LEAF POULTICE (LAURUS NOBILIS).

Ingredients: 2-3 fresh bay leaves, warm water.
Preparation: Crush the leaves, soak them in warm water and apply to the forehead.
Benefits: Natural decongestant and soothing.
Usage tips: Keep the compress on for 15-20 minutes.

28. CALENDULA FLOWER INFUSION (CALENDULA OFFICINALIS).

Ingredients: 1 teaspoon dried calendula flowers, 250 ml boiling water.
Preparation: Infuse the flowers in boiling water for 10 minutes and strain.
Benefits: Anti-inflammatory and relaxing, useful for fatigue headaches.
Usage tips: Drink hot as needed.

29. JUNIPER AND THYME ESSENTIAL OIL VAPORS.

Ingredients: 3 drops juniper essential oil, 2 drops thyme essential oil, 1 liter boiling water.
Preparation: Pour the essential oils into boiling water and breathe in the vapors.
Benefits: Stimulating and decongestant, useful for headaches related to sinusitis or colds.
Usage tips: Repeat once a day.

30. NEROLI (CITRUS AURANTIUM) ESSENTIAL OIL LOTION.

Ingredients: 3 drops neroli essential oil, 1 tablespoon carrier oil.
Preparation: Mix the oils and gently massage into the temples and forehead.
Benefits: Relaxing and soothing for emotional stress headaches.
Usage tips: Apply as needed.

31. INFUSION OF ARTICHOKE LEAVES (CYNARA SCOLYMUS).

Ingredients: 1 teaspoon dried artichoke leaves, 250 ml boiling water.
Preparation: Infuse the leaves in boiling water for 10 minutes, then strain.
Benefits: Improves circulation and relieves congestion headaches.
Usage tips: Drink hot once a day.

32. LEMON AND HOLY BASIL ESSENTIAL OIL LOTION.

Ingredients: 3 drops lemon essential oil, 2 drops holy basil essential oil, 1 teaspoon carrier oil.
Preparation: Mix the oils and gently massage the temples and nape of the neck.
Benefits: Energizing and soothing, useful for fatigue headaches.
Usage tips: Apply as needed.

33. ELM BARK (ULMUS RUBRA) DECOCTION.

Ingredients: 1 teaspoon dried elm bark, 300 ml water.
Preparation: Boil the bark in water for 15 minutes, then strain.
Benefits: Natural anti-inflammatory, reduces throbbing pain.
Usage tips: Drink once a day.

34. APPLE VINEGAR AND LAVENDER POULTICE.

Ingredients: 2 tablespoons apple cider vinegar, 1 drop lavender essential oil, one cloth.
Preparation: Mix the vinegar with the essential oil and soak a cloth. Apply to the forehead.
Benefits: Refreshing and soothing, relieves throbbing headaches.
Usage tips: Leave the compress on for 15 minutes.

35. HELICHRYSUM AND ROSEMARY VAPOR.

Ingredients: 1 teaspoon helichrysum flowers, 1 teaspoon rosemary leaves, 1 liter boiling water.
Preparation: Pour boiling water over the herbs and breathe in the vapors for 10 minutes.
Benefits: Decongestant and soothing, ideal for sinus headaches.
Usage tips: Repeat once a day.

36. ROMAN CHAMOMILE AND MARJORAM ESSENTIAL OIL LOTION.

Ingredients: 2 drops Roman chamomile essential oil, 2 drops marjoram essential oil, 1 teaspoon carrier oil.
Preparation: Mix the oils and gently massage the temples.
Benefits: Relaxing and soothing, useful for stress-related headaches.
Usage tips: Apply as needed.

37. CORIANDER SEED INFUSION (CORIANDRUM SATIVUM).

Ingredients: 1 teaspoon coriander seeds, 250 ml boiling water.
Preparation: Infuse seeds in boiling water for 10 minutes, then strain.
Benefits: Improves circulation and reduces headache pain.
Usage tips: Drink hot once a day.

38. NETTLE AND LAUREL LEAF POULTICE.

Ingredients: 2 nettle leaves, 2 bay leaves, warm water.
Preparation: Soak the leaves in warm water, crush them lightly and apply to the forehead.

Benefits: Anti-inflammatory and soothing, ideal for throbbing pains.
Usage tips: Keep for 20 minutes.

39. JASMINE AND SANDALWOOD ESSENTIAL OIL LOTION.

Ingredients: 2 drops jasmine essential oil, 2 drops sandalwood essential oil, 1 tablespoon carrier oil.
Preparation: Mix the oils and gently massage the forehead and nape of the neck.
Benefits: Relaxing and restorative, useful for headaches from mental fatigue.
Usage tips: Apply as needed.

40. HAWTHORN AND LIME BLOSSOM HERBAL TEA.

Ingredients: 1 teaspoon hawthorn flowers, 1 teaspoon linden flowers, 250 ml boiling water.
Preparation: Infuse the flowers in boiling water for 10 minutes, then strain.
Benefits: Relaxing and calming, relieves headaches from stress and insomnia.
Usage tips: Drink hot before bedtime.

SKIN CONDITIONS – NATURAL REMEDIES

This section offers natural remedies to relieve common skin ailments such as acne, irritation, eczema, and other skin issues. Each remedy is accompanied by details on ingredients, preparation, and benefits.

1. ALOE VERA (ALOE BARBADENSIS) COMPRESS.

Ingredients: 2 tablespoons of fresh aloe vera gel.
Preparation: Apply the gel directly to the affected area and leave it on for 15-20 minutes. Rinse with lukewarm water.
Benefits: Anti-inflammatory and moisturizing, useful for sunburn, irritation and dry skin.
Usage tips: Apply 2-3 times a day.

2. LAVENDER AND ROMAN CHAMOMILE ESSENTIAL OIL LOTION.

Ingredients: 3 drops lavender essential oil, 2 drops Roman chamomile essential oil, 1 tablespoon sweet almond oil.
Preparation: Mix the oils and apply to irritated skin with gentle movements.
Benefits: Soothes reddened skin and reduces inflammation.
Usage tips: Use as needed.

3. GREEN CLAY AND HONEY MASK.

Ingredients: 2 tablespoons green clay, 1 tablespoon honey, enough water.
Preparation: Mix the ingredients until you get a soft paste, apply it to the face and leave it on for 15 minutes. Rinse with lukewarm water.
Benefits: Purifies oily skin and reduces acne.
Usage tips: Apply 1-2 times a week.

4. CALENDULA FLOWER INFUSION (CALENDULA OFFICINALIS).

Ingredients: 1 tablespoon dried marigold flowers, 250 ml boiling water.
Preparation: Infuse the flowers in boiling water for 10 minutes and strain. Use the infusion as a facial tonic or compress.
Benefits: Soothing for sensitive or irritated skin.
Usage tips: Apply with a cotton ball 2 times a day.

5. TEA TREE (MELALEUCA ALTERNIFOLIA) ESSENTIAL OIL LOTION.

Ingredients: 1 drop tea tree essential oil, 1 teaspoon carrier oil.
Preparation: Mix the oils and apply directly to skin imperfections with a cotton ball.
Benefits: Antibacterial and antimicrobial, ideal for acne and pimples.
Usage tips: Use as needed, avoiding areas that are too large.

6. NETTLE LEAF DECOCTION (URTICA DIOICA).

Ingredients: 1 tablespoon dried nettle leaves, 300 ml water.
Preparation: Bring water with the leaves to a boil, simmer for 10 minutes and strain. Use the decoction as a facial tonic or wash.
Benefits: Astringent and purifying, useful for oily or acne-prone skin.
Usage tips: Apply with a cotton ball 1-2 times a day.

7. CHAMOMILE AND LINDEN POULTICE.

Ingredients: 1 teaspoon chamomile flowers, 1 teaspoon linden flowers, 250 ml boiling water.
Preparation: Prepare an infusion with the herbs, soak a clean cloth and apply it to the affected area.
Benefits: Soothing for irritation, redness and sensitive skin.
Usage tips: Use as needed.

8. TURMERIC AND YOGURT MASK.

Ingredients: 1 teaspoon turmeric powder, 2 tablespoons natural yogurt.
Preparation: Mix ingredients, apply to face and leave on for 10-15 minutes. Rinse with lukewarm water.
Benefits: Anti-inflammatory and brightening, useful for skin blemishes and dull skin.
Usage tips: Apply 1-2 times a week.

9. GERANIUM (PELARGONIUM GRAVEOLENS) ESSENTIAL OIL LOTION.

Ingredients: 3 drops geranium essential oil, 1 tablespoon jojoba oil.
Preparation: Mix the oils and apply to irritated or dry skin with gentle movements.
Benefits: Moisturizing and regenerating, it helps rebalance the skin.
Usage tips: Use as needed.

10. INFUSION OF MALLOW LEAVES (MALVA SYLVESTRIS).

Ingredients: 1 tablespoon dried mallow leaves, 250 ml boiling water.

Preparation: Infuse the leaves in boiling water for 10 minutes and strain. Use the infusion for skin washes or compresses.

Benefits: Emollient and soothing, ideal for dry or irritated skin.

Usage tips: Apply 2-3 times a day.

11. SANDALWOOD AND ROSE ESSENTIAL OIL LOTION.

Ingredients: 3 drops sandalwood essential oil, 2 drops rose essential oil, 1 tablespoon jojoba oil.

Preparation: Mix the oils and gently apply to the skin.

Benefits: Moisturizing and regenerating, useful for dry, mature skin.

Usage tips: Apply as needed, especially in the evening.

12. ROSE WATER AND OATMEAL WRAP.

Ingredients: 2 tablespoons oatmeal, enough rose water.

Preparation: Mix ingredients until a paste is obtained, apply to face and leave on for 15 minutes. Rinse with lukewarm water.

Benefits: Soothing and nourishing, ideal for irritated or reddened skin.

Usage tips: Use 1-2 times a week.

13. IVY LEAF INFUSION (HEDERA HELIX).

Ingredients: 1 teaspoon dried ivy leaves, 250 ml boiling water.

Preparation: Infuse the leaves in boiling water for 10 minutes and strain. Use the infusion for washes or compresses.

Benefits: Purifying and invigorating, useful for oily or blemish-prone skin.

Usage tips: Apply 1-2 times a day.

14. CUCUMBER AND HONEY MASK.

Ingredients: 1 cucumber, 1 tablespoon honey.

Preparation: Blend cucumber until pureed, add honey and mix. Apply to face and leave on for 15 minutes. Rinse with lukewarm water.

Benefits: Refreshing and moisturizing, reduces swelling and redness.

Usage tips: Apply 1 time per week.

15. PATCHOULI AND TEA TREE ESSENTIAL OIL LOTION.

Ingredients: 3 drops patchouli essential oil, 2 drops tea tree essential oil, 1 tablespoon coconut oil.

Preparation: Mix the oils and apply to affected areas.

Benefits: Antibacterial and healing, useful for acne and scarring.

Usage tips: Apply 1-2 times a day.

16. INFUSION OF THYME LEAVES (THYMUS VULGARIS).

Ingredients: 1 teaspoon dried thyme leaves, 250 ml boiling water.

Preparation: Infuse the leaves in boiling water for 10 minutes and strain. Use the infusion as a tonic or for washes.

Benefits: A natural antiseptic, it purifies the skin and reduces blemishes.
Usage tips: Apply 1-2 times a day.

17. AVOCADO AND ALMOND OIL MASK.

Ingredients: 1/2 ripe avocado, 1 tablespoon sweet almond oil.
Preparation: Mash the avocado and mix with the oil until smooth. Apply to face and leave on for 15 minutes. Rinse with lukewarm water.
Benefits: Nourishes and moisturizes dry, dull skin.
Usage tips: Apply 1 time per week.

18. LEMON AND LAVENDER ESSENTIAL OIL LOTION.

Ingredients: 2 drops lemon essential oil, 2 drops lavender essential oil, 1 tablespoon sweet almond oil.
Preparation: Mix the oils and apply to irritated or reddened skin.
Benefits: Soothing and invigorating, useful for tired or blotchy skin.
Usage tips: Apply 1-2 times a day.

19. BURDOCK ROOT (ARCTIUM LAPPA) DECOCTION.

Ingredients: 1 teaspoon dried burdock root, 300 ml water.
Preparation: Boil the root in water for 15 minutes, then strain. Use the decoction for washes or compresses.
Benefits: Purifying and cleansing, useful for oily or acne-prone skin.
Usage tips: Apply 1-2 times a day.

20. NEROLI AND CHAMOMILE ESSENTIAL OIL LOTION.

Ingredients: 2 drops neroli essential oil, 2 drops chamomile essential oil, 1 tablespoon jojoba oil.
Preparation: Mix the oils and apply to the skin with gentle movements.
Benefits: Regenerating and soothing, useful for dry and irritated skin.
Usage tips: Use as needed.

21. POULTICE OF MALLOW LEAVES AND CHAMOMILE.

Ingredients: 1 teaspoon dried mallow leaves, 1 teaspoon chamomile flowers, 250 ml boiling water.
Preparation: Prepare an infusion with the herbs, soak a clean cloth and apply it to irritated skin.
Benefits: Emollient and soothing, ideal for dry and reddened skin.
Usage tips: Use 2 times a day.

22. CARROT AND HONEY MASK.

Ingredients: 1 cooked and mashed carrot, 1 tablespoon honey.
Preparation: Mix ingredients until smooth, apply to face and leave on for 15 minutes. Rinse with lukewarm water.
Benefits: Nourishes and brightens skin, useful for dull or tired skin.
Usage tips: Apply 1 time per week.

23. BERGAMOT AND TEA TREE ESSENTIAL OIL LOTION.

Ingredients: 2 drops bergamot essential oil, 1 drop tea tree essential oil, 1 tablespoon coconut oil.
Preparation: Mix the oils and apply to areas with acne or blemishes.
Benefits: Antibacterial and purifying, useful for oily and acne-prone skin.
Usage tips: Use 1-2 times a day.

24. INFUSION OF VIOLA TRICOLOR FLOWERS (VIOLA TRICOLOR).

Ingredients: 1 tablespoon dried flowers of viola tricolor, 250 ml boiling water.
Preparation: Infuse the flowers in boiling water for 10 minutes and strain. Use the infusion for washes or compresses.
Benefits: Soothing and purifying, ideal for eczema and sensitive skin.
Usage tips: Apply 1-2 times a day.

25. MYRRH AND GERANIUM ESSENTIAL OIL LOTION.

Ingredients: 2 drops myrrh essential oil, 2 drops geranium essential oil, 1 tablespoon sweet almond oil.
Preparation: Mix the oils and apply to dry or cracked skin.
Benefits: Moisturizing and regenerating, useful for mature or damaged skin.
Usage tips: Use as needed.

26. HONEY AND CINNAMON MASK.

Ingredients: 1 tablespoon honey, 1/2 teaspoon cinnamon powder.
Preparation: Mix ingredients and apply to face. Leave on for 10 minutes, then rinse with lukewarm water.
Benefits: Antibacterial and purifying, ideal for acne and blemishes.
Usage tips: Apply 1 time per week.

27. RICE STARCH WRAP.

Ingredients: 2 tablespoons rice starch, enough water.
Preparation: Mix starch with water to a paste, apply to irritated area and leave on for 10-15 minutes. Rinse with lukewarm water.
Benefits: Calming and soothing, useful for itching or redness.
Usage tips: Use as needed.

28. EUCALYPTUS AND CHAMOMILE ESSENTIAL OIL LOTION.

Ingredients: 2 drops eucalyptus essential oil, 2 drops chamomile essential oil, 1 tablespoon jojoba oil.
Preparation: Mix the oils and apply to reddened or inflamed skin.
Benefits: Refreshing and soothing, useful for irritation or insect bites.
Usage tips: Apply as needed.

29. MARSHMALLOW ROOT DECOCTION (ALTHAEA OFFICINALIS).

Ingredients: 1 teaspoon dried marshmallow root, 300 ml water.

Preparation: Boil the root in water for 10 minutes, then strain. Use the decoction for washes or compresses.
Benefits: Emollient and soothing, ideal for dry, cracked skin.
Usage tips: Apply 1-2 times a day.

30. BANANA PULP AND COCONUT OIL MASK.

Ingredients: 1/2 ripe banana, 1 teaspoon coconut oil.
Preparation: Mash banana, mix with coconut oil and apply to face. Leave on for 15 minutes, then rinse with lukewarm water.
Benefits: Moisturizing and nourishing, ideal for dry, dull skin.
Usage tips: Apply once a week.

31. CYPRESS AND LAVENDER ESSENTIAL OIL LOTION.

Ingredients: 2 drops cypress essential oil, 2 drops lavender essential oil, 1 tablespoon sweet almond oil.
Preparation: Mix the oils and apply to the skin with a gentle massage.
Benefits: Soothing and invigorating, useful for sensitive or rosacea-prone skin.
Usage tips: Apply as needed.

32. BASIL AND MINT LEAF POULTICE.

Ingredients: 1 teaspoon fresh basil leaves, 1 teaspoon fresh mint leaves, 250 ml boiling water.
Preparation: Prepare an infusion with the herbs, soak a clean cloth and apply to the irritated area.
Benefits: Refreshing and cleansing, ideal for itching or redness.
Usage tips: Use 1-2 times a day.

33. TOMATO AND YOGURT MASK.

Ingredients: 1 tablespoon tomato puree, 1 tablespoon natural yogurt.
Preparation: Mix ingredients, apply to face and leave on for 15 minutes. Rinse with lukewarm water.
Benefits: Astringent and purifying, ideal for oily skin or skin with enlarged pores.
Usage tips: Apply 1 time per week.

34. SAGE AND TEA TREE ESSENTIAL OIL LOTION.

Ingredients: 2 drops sage essential oil, 2 drops tea tree essential oil, 1 tablespoon jojoba oil.
Preparation: Mix the oils and apply to imperfections.
Benefits: Purifying and healing, useful for acne and pimples.
Usage tips: Apply 1-2 times a day.

35. STRAWBERRY LEAF (FRAGARIA VESCA) DECOCTION.

Ingredients: 1 teaspoon dried strawberry leaves, 300 ml water.
Preparation: Boil the leaves in water for 10 minutes, then strain. Use the decoction for washes or compresses.
Benefits: Toning and purifying, ideal for combination or oily skin.
Usage tips: Apply as needed.

36. COCONUT WATER AND ALOE VERA WRAP.

Ingredients: 2 tablespoons aloe vera gel, 2 tablespoons coconut water.
Preparation: Mix ingredients and apply to skin with a clean cloth.
Benefits: Moisturizing and soothing, ideal for dry skin or sunburn.
Usage tips: Use 1-2 times a day.

37. CEDAR AND PATCHOULI ESSENTIAL OIL LOTION.

Ingredients: 3 drops cedar essential oil, 2 drops patchouli essential oil, 1 tablespoon sweet almond oil.
Preparation: Mix the oils and apply to the skin with a gentle massage.
Benefits: Regenerating and moisturizing, useful for dry, cracked skin.
Usage tips: Apply as needed.

38. MELON AND HONEY MASK.

Ingredients: 2 tablespoons melon puree, 1 tablespoon honey.
Preparation: Mix ingredients, apply to face and leave on for 15 minutes. Rinse with lukewarm water.
Benefits: Refreshing and moisturizing, ideal for tired or sun-exposed skin.
Usage tips: Apply 1 time per week.

39. LEMON AND BERGAMOT ESSENTIAL OIL LOTION.

Ingredients: 2 drops lemon essential oil, 2 drops bergamot essential oil, 1 tablespoon carrier oil.
Preparation: Mix the oils and apply to areas with skin spots.
Benefits: Lightening and purifying, ideal for skin spots.
Usage tips: Use in the evening to avoid sun exposure.

40. INFUSION OF DANDELION LEAVES (TARAXACUM OFFICINALE).

Ingredients: 1 tablespoon dried dandelion leaves, 250 ml boiling water.
Preparation: Infuse the leaves in boiling water for 10 minutes and strain. Use the infusion for washes or compresses.
Benefits: Purifying and invigorating, ideal for oily skin or skin with impurities.
Usage tips: Apply 1-2 times a day.

JOINT HEALTH — NATURAL REMEDIES

This section provides natural remedies to improve joint health, relieve pain, inflammation and stiffness. Each remedy is unique and offers details on ingredients, preparation, and benefits.

1. GINGER ROOT (ZINGIBER OFFICINALE) INFUSION.

Ingredients: 1 teaspoon grated fresh ginger root, 250 ml boiling water.
Preparation: Pour boiling water over ginger and let steep for 10 minutes. Strain.

Benefits: Natural anti-inflammatory, useful for reducing joint pain.
Usage tips: Drink hot 1-2 times a day.

2. ROSEMARY AND JUNIPER ESSENTIAL OIL LOTION.

Ingredients: 2 drops rosemary essential oil, 2 drops juniper essential oil, 1 tablespoon sweet almond oil.
Preparation: Mix the oils and gently massage the joints.
Benefits: Stimulates circulation and relieves joint stiffness.
Usage tips: Apply 2 times a day.

3. WILLOW BARK (SALIX ALBA) DECOCTION.

Ingredients: 1 teaspoon dried willow bark, 300 ml water.
Preparation: Boil the bark in water for 10 minutes, then strain.
Benefits: Contains salicin, a natural analgesic for joint pain.
Usage tips: Drink hot once a day.

4. GREEN CLAY AND LAVENDER ESSENTIAL OIL POULTICE.

Ingredients: 2 tablespoons green clay, 1 drop lavender essential oil, water as needed.
Preparation: Mix clay with water to a paste, add essential oil and apply to aching joints. Leave on for 20 minutes, then rinse.
Benefits: Reduces inflammation and pain.
Usage tips: Use as needed.

5. ARNICA AND CHAMOMILE ESSENTIAL OIL LOTION.

Ingredients: 3 drops arnica essential oil, 2 drops chamomile essential oil, 1 tablespoon carrier oil (e.g., almond oil).
Preparation: Mix the oils and apply with gentle massage to the joints.
Benefits: Anti-inflammatory and relaxing, reduces stiffness.
Usage tips: Apply 1-2 times a day.

6. TURMERIC AND BLACK PEPPER INFUSION (CURCUMA LONGA AND PIPER NIGRUM).

Ingredients: 1 teaspoon turmeric powder, a pinch of black pepper, 250 ml boiling water.
Preparation: Pour boiling water over turmeric and pepper, stir and let steep for 5 minutes.
Benefits: Reduces inflammation and supports joint mobility.
Usage tips: Drink hot once a day.

7. CABBAGE LEAF POULTICE.

Ingredients: 2-3 fresh cabbage leaves.
Preparation: Lightly crush the leaves to release the juice and apply to the joints, covering with gauze.
Benefits: Natural anti-inflammatory, relieves swelling and pain.
Usage tips: Keep the compress on for 20-30 minutes, 1 time a day.

8. WINTERGREEN AND MINT ESSENTIAL OIL LOTION.

Ingredients: 2 drops wintergreen essential oil, 2 drops peppermint essential oil, 1 tablespoon carrier oil.
Preparation: Mix the oils and apply to the joints with a massage.
Benefits: Pain-relieving and cooling, useful for stiff joints.
Usage tips: Apply as needed.

9. BURDOCK ROOT (ARCTIUM LAPPA) DECOCTION.

Ingredients: 1 teaspoon dried burdock root, 300 ml water.
Preparation: Boil the root in water for 10 minutes, then strain.
Benefits: Natural depurative, helps reduce toxin-related joint pain.
Usage tips: Drink once a day.

10. EUCALYPTUS AND ARNICA ESSENTIAL OIL LOTION.

Ingredients: 2 drops eucalyptus essential oil, 2 drops arnica essential oil, 1 tablespoon coconut oil.
Preparation: Mix the oils and apply to the joints with gentle movements.
Benefits: Stimulates circulation and relieves muscle and joint pain.
Usage tips: Use 1-2 times a day.

11. INFUSION OF NETTLE LEAVES (URTICA DIOICA)

Ingredients: 1 tablespoon dried nettle leaves, 250 ml boiling water.
Preparation: Infuse the leaves in boiling water for 10 minutes and strain.
Benefits: Anti-inflammatory and depurative, useful for reducing joint pain.
Usage tips: Drink hot once a day.

12. GINGER AND BLACK PEPPER ESSENTIAL OIL LOTION.

Ingredients: 2 drops ginger essential oil, 1 drop black pepper essential oil, 1 tablespoon sweet almond oil.
Preparation: Mix the oils and gently massage the joints.
Benefits: Warming and anti-inflammatory, relieves joint stiffness.
Usage tips: Apply 1-2 times a day.

13. BIRCH LEAF (BETULA PENDULA) DECOCTION.

Ingredients: 1 tablespoon dried birch leaves, 300 ml water.
Preparation: Bring water to a boil with the leaves, simmer for 10 minutes and strain.
Benefits: Purifying and draining, reduces joint inflammation.
Usage tips: Drink once a day.

14. CASTOR OIL AND TURMERIC POULTICE.

Ingredients: 2 tablespoons castor oil, 1 teaspoon turmeric powder.
Preparation: Mix ingredients, apply to joints and cover with gauze. Leave on for 20 to 30 minutes.

Benefits: Natural anti-inflammatory and pain reliever.
Usage tips: Use as needed.

15. BASIL AND LAVENDER ESSENTIAL OIL LOTION.

Ingredients: 3 drops basil essential oil, 2 drops lavender essential oil, 1 tablespoon carrier oil.
Preparation: Mix the oils and massage the joints in circular motions.
Benefits: Relaxing and anti-inflammatory, ideal for mild pain.
Usage tips: Apply 1-2 times a day.

16. ELDERFLOWER (SAMBUCUS NIGRA) INFUSION.

Ingredients: 1 tablespoon dried elderberry flowers, 250 ml boiling water.
Preparation: Infuse the flowers in boiling water for 10 minutes and strain.
Benefits: Promotes circulation and relieves inflammation.
Usage tips: Drink once a day.

17. MYRTLE AND ROSEMARY ESSENTIAL OIL LOTION.

Ingredients: 2 drops myrtle essential oil, 2 drops rosemary essential oil, 1 tablespoon sweet almond oil.
Preparation: Mix the oils and massage into the joints.
Benefits: Stimulates circulation and relieves stiffness pain.
Usage tips: Apply as needed.

18. LICORICE ROOT (GLYCYRRHIZA GLABRA) DECOCTION.

Ingredients: 1 tablespoon dried licorice root, 300 ml water.
Preparation: Boil the root in water for 10 minutes and strain.
Benefits: Natural anti-inflammatory, useful for reducing chronic joint pain.
Usage tips: Drink hot once a day.

19. LAUREL LEAF AND OLIVE OIL POULTICE.

Ingredients: 3 bay leaves, 2 tablespoons olive oil.
Preparation: Lightly crush the leaves, dip them in the oil and warm slightly. Apply to joints with gauze.
Benefits: Soothing and anti-inflammatory, reduces swelling and pain.
Usage tips: Use as needed.

20. CYPRESS AND WINTERGREEN ESSENTIAL OIL LOTION.

Ingredients: 2 drops cypress essential oil, 2 drops wintergreen essential oil, 1 tablespoon carrier oil.
Preparation: Mix the oils and gently massage the joints.
Benefits: Relieves pain and improves joint mobility.
Usage tips: Apply 1-2 times a day.

21. FENNEL SEED INFUSION (FOENICULUM VULGARE)

Ingredients: 1 teaspoon fennel seeds, 250 ml boiling water.
Preparation: Pour boiling water over the seeds and let steep for 10 minutes. Strain.
Benefits: Helps reduce inflammation and improves circulation.
Usage tips: Drink once a day.

22. LEMONGRASS AND JUNIPER ESSENTIAL OIL LOTION.

Ingredients: 2 drops lemongrass essential oil, 2 drops juniper essential oil, 1 tablespoon sweet almond oil.
Preparation: Mix the oils and apply by massage to the joints.
Benefits: Invigorating and pain-relieving, relieves joint stiffness.
Usage tips: Use 1-2 times a day.

23. ASH (FRAXINUS EXCELSIOR) BARK DECOCTION.

Ingredients: 1 teaspoon dried bark, 300 ml water.
Preparation: Boil the bark in water for 15 minutes, then strain.
Benefits: Depurative and anti-inflammatory, useful for chronic joint pain.
Usage tips: Drink hot once a day.

24. BIRCH LEAF AND ROSE WATER POULTICE.

Ingredients: 2 birch leaves, 2 tablespoons rose water.
Preparation: Lightly crush the leaves, soak them in rose water and apply to the joints with gauze.
Benefits: Soothing and anti-inflammatory, ideal for swollen joints.
Usage tips: Use as needed.

25. PEPPERMINT AND CLOVE ESSENTIAL OIL LOTION.

Ingredients: 2 drops peppermint essential oil, 2 drops clove essential oil, 1 tablespoon carrier oil.
Preparation: Mix the oils and apply to the joints with gentle massage.
Benefits: Refreshing and pain-relieving, reduces muscle tension.
Usage tips: Apply as needed.

26. INFUSION OF HORSETAIL LEAVES (EQUISETUM ARVENSE).

Ingredients: 1 tablespoon dried horsetail leaves, 250 ml boiling water.
Preparation: Infuse the leaves in boiling water for 10 minutes and strain.
Benefits: Rich in minerals, supports joint regeneration.
Usage tips: Drink once a day.

27. LAVENDER AND WINTERGREEN ESSENTIAL OIL LOTION.

Ingredients: 2 drops lavender essential oil, 2 drops wintergreen essential oil, 1 tablespoon coconut oil.
Preparation: Mix the oils and apply with gentle movements to the joints.

Benefits: Relaxing and anti-inflammatory, ideal for muscle and joint pain.
Usage tips: Apply 1-2 times a day.

28. DANDELION ROOT DECOCTION (TARAXACUM OFFICINALE).

Ingredients: 1 tablespoon dried dandelion root, 300 ml water.
Preparation: Boil the root in water for 10 minutes and strain.
Benefits: Depurative and anti-inflammatory, useful for joint pain caused by toxin buildup.
Usage tips: Drink once a day.

29. WHITE CLAY AND TEA TREE OIL POULTICE.

Ingredients: 2 tablespoons white clay, 2 drops tea tree essential oil, water as needed.
Preparation: Mix clay with water and essential oil to a paste, apply to joints and leave on for 20 minutes.
Benefits: Purifying and anti-inflammatory, reduces swelling.
Usage tips: Use as needed.

30. ROSEMARY AND CEDAR ESSENTIAL OIL LOTION.

Ingredients: 2 drops rosemary essential oil, 2 drops cedar essential oil, 1 tablespoon carrier oil.
Preparation: Mix the oils and gently massage into the joints.
Benefits: Stimulates circulation and relieves joint pain.
Usage tips: Apply 1-2 times a day.

31. ANISEED INFUSION (PIMPINELLA ANISUM)

Ingredients: 1 teaspoon anise seeds, 250 ml boiling water.
Preparation: Pour boiling water over the seeds and let steep for 10 minutes. Strain.
Benefits: Anti-inflammatory and soothing, useful for mild joint pain.
Usage tips: Drink once a day.

32. SCOTS PINE AND LAVENDER ESSENTIAL OIL LOTION.

Ingredients: 2 drops Scots pine essential oil, 2 drops lavender essential oil, 1 tablespoon sweet almond oil.
Preparation: Mix the oils and gently massage the joints.
Benefits: Relaxing and anti-inflammatory, relieves muscle and joint pain.
Usage tips: Apply as needed.

33. JUNIPER LEAF (JUNIPERUS COMMUNIS) DECOCTION.

Ingredients: 1 tablespoon dried juniper leaves, 300 ml water.
Preparation: Boil the leaves in water for 10 minutes, then strain.
Benefits: Natural depurative, reduces toxin buildup in joints.
Usage tips: Drink once a day.

34. LAUREL LEAF AND LEMON ESSENTIAL OIL POULTICE.

Ingredients: 2 bay leaves, 2 drops of lemon essential oil, warm water.
Preparation: Soak leaves in warm water, add essential oil and apply to joints with gauze.
Benefits: Soothing and stimulating, relieves joint swelling.
Usage tips: Keep the compress on for 20-30 minutes.

35. CINNAMON AND WINTERGREEN ESSENTIAL OIL LOTION.

Ingredients: 1 drop cinnamon essential oil, 2 drops wintergreen essential oil, 1 tablespoon coconut oil.
Preparation: Mix the oils and apply with a gentle massage.
Benefits: Warming and pain-relieving, reduces joint stiffness.
Usage tips: Apply as needed.

36. HAWTHORN (CRATAEGUS MONOGYNA) FLOWER INFUSION.

Ingredients: 1 tablespoon dried hawthorn flowers, 250 ml boiling water.
Preparation: Infuse the flowers in boiling water for 10 minutes and strain.
Benefits: Promotes circulation and reduces joint pain related to poor circulation.
Usage tips: Drink once a day.

37. YLANG YLANG AND GINGER ESSENTIAL OIL LOTION.

Ingredients: 2 drops ylang ylang essential oil, 1 drop ginger essential oil, 1 tablespoon carrier oil.
Preparation: Mix the oils and gently massage the joints.
Benefits: Relaxing and anti-inflammatory, relieves muscle tension.
Usage tips: Apply 1-2 times a day.

38. DECOCTION OF ENULA CAMPANA ROOT (INULA HELENIUM).

Ingredients: 1 tablespoon dried enula campana root, 300 ml water.
Preparation: Boil the root in water for 10 minutes and strain.
Benefits: Natural anti-inflammatory, useful for chronic joint pain.
Usage tips: Drink once a day.

39. SESAME SEED OIL AND TURMERIC POULTICE.

Ingredients: 2 tablespoons sesame seed oil, 1 teaspoon turmeric powder.
Preparation: Mix ingredients and apply to joints with gauze.
Benefits: Moisturizing and anti-inflammatory, relieves swelling and stiffness.
Usage tips: Use as needed.

40. EUCALYPTUS AND SAGE ESSENTIAL OIL LOTION.

Ingredients: 2 drops eucalyptus essential oil, 2 drops sage essential oil, 1 tablespoon sweet almond oil.
Preparation: Mix the oils and apply by massage to the joints.

Benefits: Stimulates circulation and reduces joint stiffness.
Usage tips: Apply 1-2 times a day.

41. MAGNESIUM SALTS BATH

Ingredients: 2 cups Epsom salts (magnesium sulfate), hot water.
Preparation: Dissolve the salts in a tub of hot water and soak for 20-30 minutes.
Benefits: Relaxes muscles, relieves joint stiffness and reduces inflammation.
Usage tips: Take the bath 1-2 times a week.

42. BATH WITH EPSOM SALTS AND LAVENDER ESSENTIAL OIL.

Ingredients: 2 cups Epsom salts, 5 drops lavender essential oil, hot water.
Preparation: Dissolve the salts and add the essential oil to a tub of warm water. Soak for 20 to 30 minutes.
Benefits: Calming and anti-inflammatory, relieves joint and muscle pain.
Usage tips: Use as needed, preferably in the evening.

43. BATH WITH HIMALAYAN SALTS AND ROSEMARY OIL.
Ingredients: 2 cups Himalayan pink salts, 5 drops rosemary essential oil, hot water.
Preparation: Dissolve the salts and add the oil in hot water. Soak for 20 minutes.
Benefits: Invigorating and soothing for joint pain.
Usage tips: Bathe once a week.

44. GREEN CLAY AND EPSOM SALTS BATH.

Ingredients: 1 cup green clay powder, 1 cup Epsom salts, hot water.
Preparation: Mix the ingredients in the hot water in the bath and soak for 20 minutes.
Benefits: Purifying and anti-inflammatory, useful for joint swelling.
Usage tips: Bathe as needed.

45. EPSOM SALTS AND HOT WATER WRAP.

Ingredients: 1 cup of Epsom salts, warm water, a clean cloth.
Preparation: Dissolve the salts in hot water, dip a cloth in the solution and apply it to sore joints.
Benefits: Soothes and reduces inflammation.
Usage tips: Apply as needed for 15-20 minutes.

46. FOOT BATH WITH MAGNESIUM SALTS AND MINT OIL.

Ingredients: 1 cup Epsom salts, 5 drops of mint essential oil, warm water.
Preparation: Dissolve the salts and essential oil in a basin of warm water. Soak the feet for 15 to 20 minutes.
Benefits: Relieves joint pain in the feet and improves circulation.
Usage tips: Make as needed.

47. BATH WITH SODIUM BAKING SODA AND CHAMOMILE ESSENTIAL OIL.

Ingredients: 1 cup baking soda, 5 drops chamomile essential oil, warm water.
Preparation: Mix the baking soda and essential oil in the hot water in the bath. Soak for 20 minutes.
Benefits: Relaxing and detoxifying, relieves joint pain.
Usage tips: Take the bath once a week.

48. BATH WITH SEA SALT AND EUCALYPTUS ESSENTIAL OIL.

Ingredients: 2 cups sea salt, 5 drops eucalyptus essential oil, hot water.
Preparation: Dissolve the salts and add the oil to the hot water. Soak for 20 minutes.
Benefits: Decongestant and pain-relieving, useful for stiff joints.
Usage tips: Use as needed.

49. FOOT BATH WITH HIMALAYAN SALT AND TURMERIC.

Ingredients: 1 cup Himalayan pink salt, 1 teaspoon turmeric powder, hot water.
Preparation: Mix ingredients in a bowl of hot water and soak feet for 15-20 minutes.
Benefits: Anti-inflammatory and stimulating for the joints of the feet.
Usage tips: Make as needed.

50. BATH WITH CHAMOMILE FLOWERS AND EPSOM SALTS.

Ingredients: 1 cup Epsom salts, 1 cup dried chamomile flowers, hot water.
Preparation: Pour the salts and flowers into the hot water in the tub and soak for 20-30 minutes.
Benefits: Soothing and relaxing, reduces muscle and joint pain.
Usage tips: Take the bath 1-2 times a week.

CHAPTER 9:
REMEDIES FOR MENTAL HEALTH AND WELL-BEING

Mental health is an essential part of overall well-being, influencing how we live, work and face daily challenges. A balanced mental state contributes to greater resilience, better stress management and a more peaceful quality of life. This chapter presents natural remedies and simple strategies to support calmness, improve mood and promote relaxation.

Through the use of calming herbs, breathing techniques and lifestyle changes, you will discover effective ways to manage anxiety, insomnia and mental fatigue. These remedies are designed to integrate easily into your routine, offering long-term support and promoting a feeling of balance and serenity.

Begin your journey to more stable mental well-being with practical and natural solutions that respect the rhythms of your body and mind.

STRESS AND ANXIETY — NATURAL REMEDIES

This section presents a variety of natural remedies for dealing with stress and anxiety, helping you regain calm and focus. Each remedy is designed to be easily integrated into your daily routine, promoting lasting mental well-being.

1. LEMON BALM INFUSION (MELISSA OFFICINALIS)

Ingredients: 1 teaspoon dried lemon balm leaves, 250 ml boiling water.
Preparation: Pour boiling water over the leaves and let steep for 10 minutes. Strain.
Benefits: Calming and relaxing, helps reduce anxiety and stress.
Usage tips: Drink one cup as needed, up to 2 times a day.

2. LAVENDER ESSENTIAL OIL LOTION.

Ingredients: 3 drops lavender essential oil, 1 tablespoon sweet almond oil.
Preparation: Mix the oils and gently massage the temples and nape of the neck.
Benefits: Relaxes the mind and reduces symptoms of stress.
Usage tips: Use as needed, preferably before bedtime.

3. BATH WITH MAGNESIUM AND CHAMOMILE SALTS.

Ingredients: 2 cups Epsom salts, 1 cup dried chamomile flowers, hot water.
Preparation: Add the salts and flowers to the hot water in the bath and soak for 20-30 minutes.
Benefits: Soothing and relaxing, relieves muscle tension and mental stress.
Usage tips: Take the bath 1-2 times a week.

THE ART OF HOME APOTHECARY

4. LIME TREE HERBAL TEA (TILIA CORDATA).

Ingredients: 1 teaspoon linden flowers, 250 ml boiling water.
Preparation: Infuse the flowers in boiling water for 10 minutes and strain.
Benefits: Relaxing and calming, ideal for states of agitation.
Usage tips: Drink hot as needed, up to 2 times a day.

5. YLANG YLANG AND BERGAMOT ESSENTIAL OIL LOTION.

Ingredients: 2 drops ylang ylang essential oil, 2 drops bergamot essential oil, 1 tablespoon jojoba oil.
Preparation: Mix the oils and apply with gentle massage to the solar plexus.
Benefits: Reduces tension and promotes inner calm.
Usage tips: Apply as needed.

6. PASSIONFLOWER (PASSIFLORA INCARNATA) INFUSION.

Ingredients: 1 teaspoon dried passion flower leaves, 250 ml boiling water.
Preparation: Pour boiling water over the leaves, let steep for 10 minutes and strain.
Benefits: Reduces anxiety and promotes relaxation.
Usage tips: Drink one cup before bedtime.

7. WRAP WITH CHAMOMILE OIL AND WHITE CLAY.

Ingredients: 2 tablespoons white clay, 1 tablespoon chamomile oil, enough water.
Preparation: Mix the ingredients until you get a paste and apply to the shoulders or nape of the neck. Leave on for 15 minutes.
Benefits: Relaxes muscles and relieves tension caused by stress.
Usage tips: Use as needed.

8. CEDAR AND LAVENDER ESSENTIAL OIL LOTION.

Ingredients: 2 drops cedar essential oil, 2 drops lavender essential oil, 1 tablespoon coconut oil.
Preparation: Mix the oils and gently massage the feet.
Benefits: Promotes relaxation and grounding, useful for times of intense anxiety.
Usage tips: Apply before bedtime.

9. VALERIAN HERBAL TEA (VALERIANA OFFICINALIS).

Ingredients: 1 teaspoon dried valerian root, 250 ml boiling water.
Preparation: Infuse the root in boiling water for 10 minutes and strain.
Benefits: Calming and relaxing, useful for anxiety and insomnia.
Usage tips: Drink one cup before bedtime.

10. SWEET ORANGE AND TANGERINE ESSENTIAL OIL LOTION.

Ingredients: 3 drops sweet orange essential oil, 2 drops tangerine essential oil, 1 tablespoon carrier oil.

Preparation: Mix the oils and massage the solar plexus in circular motions.
Benefits: Stimulates good mood and reduces stress.
Usage tips: Apply as needed.

11. HAWTHORN FLOWER INFUSION (CRATAEGUS MONOGYNA).

Ingredients: 1 tablespoon dried hawthorn flowers, 250 ml boiling water.
Preparation: Pour boiling water over the flowers and let steep for 10 minutes. Strain.
Benefits: Promotes relaxation and reduces anxiety-related tachycardia.
Usage tips: Drink one cup 1-2 times a day.

12. ROSE AND CHAMOMILE ESSENTIAL OIL LOTION.

Ingredients: 2 drops rose essential oil, 2 drops chamomile essential oil, 1 tablespoon jojoba oil.
Preparation: Mix the oils and gently massage the temples and neck.
Benefits: Relaxes the mind and promotes a sense of inner calm.
Usage tips: Use as needed.

13. MALLOW AND LIME TREE LEAF POULTICE.

Ingredients: 1 tablespoon dried mallow leaves, 1 tablespoon linden flowers, 250 ml boiling water.
Preparation: Prepare an infusion with the herbs, soak a clean cloth and apply it to the forehead or solar plexus.
Benefits: Soothes agitation and reduces stress.
Usage tips: Use as needed.

14. BATH WITH OAT MILK AND LAVENDER OIL.

Ingredients: 1 cup oat milk, 5 drops lavender essential oil, warm water.
Preparation: Add the oat milk and essential oil to the warm water in the tub and soak for 20-30 minutes.
Benefits: Hydrates skin, relaxes muscles and calms the mind.
Usage tips: Take the bath 1 time a week.

15. VERBENA LEAF HERBAL TEA (ALOYSIA CITRODORA).

Ingredients: 1 teaspoon dried verbena leaves, 250 ml boiling water.
Preparation: Infuse the leaves in boiling water for 10 minutes and strain.
Benefits: Promotes relaxation and reduces symptoms of mild anxiety.
Usage tips: Drink one cup as needed.

16. GERANIUM AND SWEET ORANGE ESSENTIAL OIL LOTION.

Ingredients: 2 drops geranium essential oil, 2 drops sweet orange essential oil, 1 tablespoon sweet almond oil.
Preparation: Mix the oils and apply with a massage to the solar plexus and wrists.
Benefits: Promotes a sense of tranquility and well-being.
Usage tips: Use as needed.

17. ELDERFLOWER (SAMBUCUS NIGRA) INFUSION.

Ingredients: 1 teaspoon dried elderflowers, 250 ml boiling water.
Preparation: Pour boiling water over the flowers and let steep for 10 minutes. Strain.
Benefits: Relaxing and calming, ideal for mild nervous tension.
Usage tips: Drink one cup before bedtime.

18. PEPPERMINT AND YLANG YLANG ESSENTIAL OIL LOTION.

Ingredients: 2 drops peppermint essential oil, 2 drops ylang ylang essential oil, 1 tablespoon carrier oil.
Preparation: Mix the oils and apply in circular motions to the nape of the neck and shoulders.
Benefits: Relieves muscle and mental tension.
Usage tips: Apply 1-2 times a day.

19. FOOT BATH WITH SEA SALT AND CHAMOMILE

Ingredients: 1 cup sea salt, 1 tablespoon dried chamomile flowers, warm water.
Preparation: Mix ingredients in a bowl of warm water and soak feet for 15-20 minutes.
Benefits: Relaxes the body and promotes a general sense of calm.
Usage tips: Make as needed.

20. SANDALWOOD AND NEROLI ESSENTIAL OIL LOTION.

Ingredients: 2 drops sandalwood essential oil, 2 drops neroli essential oil, 1 tablespoon carrier oil.
Preparation: Mix the oils and massage into the solar plexus and wrists.
Benefits: Promotes serenity and reduces symptoms of anxiety.
Usage tips: Use as needed, preferably before bedtime.

21. INFUSION OF SACRED BASIL LEAVES (TULSI)

Ingredients: 1 teaspoon dried holy basil leaves, 250 ml boiling water.
Preparation: Pour boiling water over the leaves, let steep for 10 minutes and strain.
Benefits: Natural adaptogen, helps reduce cortisol levels and stress.
Usage tips: Drink one cup daily, preferably in the morning.

22. VETIVER AND ROMAN CHAMOMILE ESSENTIAL OIL LOTION.

Ingredients: 2 drops vetiver essential oil, 2 drops Roman chamomile essential oil, 1 tablespoon jojoba oil.
Preparation: Mix the oils and massage into the solar plexus and nape of the neck.
Benefits: Promotes calm and reduces deep anxiety.
Usage tips: Apply 1-2 times a day.

23. BATH WITH WHITE CLAY AND ROSE OIL.

Ingredients: 1 cup white clay, 5 drops rose essential oil, warm water.
Preparation: Dissolve the clay and essential oil in the hot water of the bath and soak for 20 minutes.

Chapter 9: Remedies for Mental Health and Well-Being

Benefits: Soothing to the mind and relaxing to the body.
Usage tips: Take the bath once a week.

24. HERBAL TEA OF HORSETAIL LEAVES (EQUISETUM ARVENSE).

Ingredients: 1 teaspoon dried horsetail leaves, 250 ml boiling water.
Preparation: Infuse the leaves in boiling water for 10 minutes and strain.
Benefits: Natural tonic for the nervous system, helps calm the mind.
Usage tips: Drink 1-2 cups a day.

25. BERGAMOT AND CEDAR ESSENTIAL OIL LOTION.

Ingredients: 2 drops bergamot essential oil, 2 drops cedar essential oil, 1 tablespoon carrier oil.
Preparation: Mix oils and gently massage into wrists and neck.
Benefits: Stimulates a sense of serenity and reduces nervousness.
Usage tips: Apply as needed.

26. OAT MILK AND LIME BLOSSOM FOOT BATH.

Ingredients: 1 cup oat milk, 2 tablespoons dried linden blossoms, warm water.
Preparation: Mix ingredients in a bowl of warm water and soak feet for 15 minutes.
Benefits: Calms nerves and relaxes the body.
Usage tips: Make as needed, preferably in the evening.

27. LEMONGRASS AND SANDALWOOD ESSENTIAL OIL LOTION.

Ingredients: 2 drops lemongrass essential oil, 2 drops sandalwood essential oil, 1 tablespoon coconut oil.
Preparation: Mix the oils and apply with a massage to the nape of the neck and chest.
Benefits: Energizing and calming, reduces tension.
Usage tips: Use 1-2 times a day.

28. CORIANDER SEED INFUSION (CORIANDRUM SATIVUM).

Ingredients: 1 teaspoon coriander seeds, 250 ml boiling water.
Preparation: Infuse seeds in boiling water for 10 minutes and strain.
Benefits: Promotes relaxation and reduces mild stress.
Usage tips: Drink 1 cup daily.

29. NEROLI AND ROSEMARY ESSENTIAL OIL LOTION.

Ingredients: 2 drops neroli essential oil, 1 drop rosemary essential oil, 1 tablespoon carrier oil.
Preparation: Mix the oils and gently massage the wrists and solar plexus.
Benefits: Promotes calmness and improves mental focus.
Usage tips: Use as needed.

THE ART OF HOME APOTHECARY

30. BATH WITH HIMALAYAN PINK SALT AND TANGERINE ESSENTIAL OIL.

Ingredients: 2 cups of pink salt, 5 drops of tangerine essential oil, hot water.
Preparation: Dissolve the salts and oil in the hot water of the bath and soak for 20-30 minutes.
Benefits: Reduces tension and promotes a sense of mental lightness.
Usage tips: Take the bath 1-2 times a week.

31. LICORICE ROOT (GLYCYRRHIZA GLABRA) INFUSION.

Ingredients: 1 teaspoon dried licorice root, 250 ml boiling water.
Preparation: Infuse the root in boiling water for 10 minutes and strain.
Benefits: Natural adaptogen, helps reduce symptoms of stress and mental fatigue.
Usage tips: Drink one cup a day.

32. PALMAROSA AND BITTER ORANGE ESSENTIAL OIL LOTION.

Ingredients: 2 drops palmarosa essential oil, 2 drops bitter orange essential oil, 1 tablespoon sweet almond oil.
Preparation: Mix the oils and massage into the solar plexus and nape of the neck.
Benefits: Reduces stress and promotes an overall sense of well-being.
Usage tips: Apply as needed.

33. BASIL AND CHAMOMILE LEAF POULTICE.

Ingredients: 1 tablespoon fresh basil leaves, 1 tablespoon chamomile flowers, 250 ml boiling water.
Preparation: Prepare an infusion with the herbs, soak a clean cloth and apply to the forehead.
Benefits: Calms the mind and reduces nervous tension.
Usage tips: Use as needed.

34. LAVENDER FLOWER AND ALMOND MILK BATH.

Ingredients: 1 cup almond milk, 5 tablespoons dried lavender flowers, hot water.
Preparation: Mix the milk and flowers in the tub of hot water and soak for 20 minutes.
Benefits: Moisturizing and relaxing, promotes muscle and mental relaxation.
Usage tips: Take the bath once a week.

35. LEMON BALM AND PEPPERMINT ESSENTIAL OIL LOTION.

Ingredients: 2 drops of lemon balm essential oil, 2 drops of peppermint essential oil, 1 tablespoon of carrier oil.
Preparation: Mix the oils and gently massage the nape of the neck and shoulders.
Benefits: Refreshing and soothing, reduces tension.
Usage tips: Apply as needed.

36. ANGELICA ROOT HERBAL TEA (ANGELICA ARCHANGELICA).

Ingredients: 1 teaspoon dried angelica root, 250 ml boiling water.
Preparation: Infuse the root in boiling water for 10 minutes and strain.

Benefits: Adaptogen that promotes relaxation and reduces stress.
Usage tips: Drink one cup daily.

37. LEMONGRASS AND ROSE ESSENTIAL OIL LOTION.

Ingredients: 2 drops lemongrass essential oil, 2 drops rose essential oil, 1 tablespoon coconut oil.
Preparation: Mix the oils and apply with a massage to the temples and neck.
Benefits: Stimulates calmness and relieves mental fatigue.
Usage tips: Use as needed.

38. FOOT BATH WITH WHITE CLAY AND EPSOM SALT.

Ingredients: 1 cup white clay, 1 cup Epsom salt, hot water.
Preparation: Dissolve ingredients in a bowl of warm water and soak feet for 15-20 minutes.
Benefits: Relaxes muscles and promotes general relaxation.
Usage tips: Make as needed.

39. CYPRESS AND LAVENDER ESSENTIAL OIL LOTION.

Ingredients: 2 drops cypress essential oil, 2 drops lavender essential oil, 1 tablespoon carrier oil.
Preparation: Mix the oils and gently massage the solar plexus and shoulders.
Benefits: Promotes deep relaxation and reduces muscle tension.
Usage tips: Apply 1-2 times a day.

40. BATH WITH SEA SALT AND YLANG YLANG ESSENTIAL OIL.

Ingredients: 2 cups sea salt, 5 drops ylang ylang essential oil, warm water.
Preparation: Dissolve the salt and oil in the hot water of the bath and soak for 20 minutes.
Benefits: Relaxes the mind and promotes inner calm.
Usage tips: Take the bath 1-2 times a week.

RESTFUL SLEEP – NATURAL REMEDIES

Quality sleep is essential for mental and physical well-being. This section offers natural remedies to promote deep, restorative sleep, helping you relax and wake up full of energy.

1. CHAMOMILE (MATRICARIA CHAMOMILLA) INFUSION.

Ingredients: 1 tablespoon dried chamomile flowers, 250 ml boiling water.
Preparation: Pour boiling water over the flowers and let steep for 10 minutes. Strain.
Benefits: Calming and relaxing, helps promote sleep.
Usage tips: Drink one cup before bedtime.

2. LAVENDER ESSENTIAL OIL LOTION.

Ingredients: 3 drops lavender essential oil, 1 tablespoon sweet almond oil.
Preparation: Mix the oils and gently massage the temples, neck and wrists.
Benefits: Promotes relaxation and calms the mind, ideal for aiding sleep.
Usage tips: Apply every night before bedtime.

3. BATH WITH MAGNESIUM SALTS AND NEROLI OIL.

Ingredients: 2 cups Epsom salts, 5 drops neroli essential oil, warm water.
Preparation: Dissolve the salts and oil in the hot water of the bath and soak for 20-30 minutes.
Benefits: Relaxes the body and calms the mind, promoting deep sleep.
Usage tips: Take the bath 1-2 times a week.

4. VALERIAN (VALERIANA OFFICINALIS) HERBAL TEA.

Ingredients: 1 teaspoon dried valerian root, 250 ml boiling water.
Preparation: Infuse the root in boiling water for 10 minutes and strain.
Benefits: Natural relaxant and sedative, helps with insomnia.
Usage tips: Drink one cup half an hour before bedtime.

5. YLANG YLANG AND SANDALWOOD ESSENTIAL OIL LOTION.

Ingredients: 2 drops ylang ylang essential oil, 2 drops sandalwood essential oil, 1 tablespoon carrier oil.
Preparation: Mix the oils and massage into the solar plexus and wrists.
Benefits: Promotes deep relaxation and peaceful sleep.
Usage tips: Apply as needed, preferably in the evening.

6. LIME TREE (TILIA CORDATA) INFUSION.

Ingredients: 1 tablespoon linden flowers, 250 ml boiling water.
Preparation: Infuse the flowers in boiling water for 10 minutes and strain.
Benefits: Calming and relaxing, useful for aiding sleep.
Usage tips: Drink one cup before bedtime.

7. CEDAR AND LAVENDER ESSENTIAL OIL LOTION.

Ingredients: 2 drops cedar essential oil, 2 drops lavender essential oil, 1 tablespoon sweet almond oil.
Preparation: Mix the oils and gently massage feet and neck.
Benefits: Relaxes the body and prepares the mind for sleep.
Usage tips: Apply every evening.

8. FOOTBATH WITH ROSE WATER AND SEA SALT.

Ingredients: 1 cup sea salt, 2 tablespoons rose water, warm water.
Preparation: Mix ingredients in a bowl of warm water and soak feet for 15 minutes.

Benefits: Calms nerves and relaxes the body.
Usage tips: Make every night before bedtime.

9. LAVENDER AND CHAMOMILE FLOWER HERBAL TEA.

Ingredients: 1 teaspoon lavender flowers, 1 teaspoon chamomile flowers, 250 ml boiling water.
Preparation: Infuse the herbs in boiling water for 10 minutes and strain.
Benefits: Soothing and calming, promotes peaceful sleep.
Usage tips: Drink one cup before bedtime.

10. NEROLI AND BERGAMOT ESSENTIAL OIL LOTION.

Ingredients: 2 drops neroli essential oil, 2 drops bergamot essential oil, 1 tablespoon carrier oil.
Preparation: Mix the oils and gently massage the temples and solar plexus.
Benefits: Promotes mental and physical relaxation.
Usage tips: Apply every night before bedtime.

11. HAWTHORN FLOWER INFUSION (CRATAEGUS MONOGYNA).

Ingredients: 1 tablespoon dried hawthorn flowers, 250 ml boiling water.
Preparation: Pour boiling water over the flowers and let steep for 10 minutes. Strain.
Benefits: Calming to the nervous system, helps to relax and aid sleep.
Usage tips: Drink one cup before bedtime.

12. PALMAROSA AND ROSE ESSENTIAL OIL LOTION.

Ingredients: 2 drops palmarosa essential oil, 2 drops rose essential oil, 1 tablespoon sweet almond oil.
Preparation: Mix the oils and gently massage the solar plexus and temples.
Benefits: Promotes a sense of peace and promotes restorative sleep.
Usage tips: Apply as needed.

13. BATH WITH CHAMOMILE FLOWERS AND OAT MILK.

Ingredients: 1 cup oat milk, 5 tablespoons dried chamomile flowers, hot water.
Preparation: Mix the milk and flowers in the tub of hot water and soak for 20 minutes.
Benefits: Hydrates and relaxes the body, improving sleep quality.
Usage tips: Take the bath once a week.

14. VIOLA TRICOLOR FLOWER HERBAL TEA (VIOLA TRICOLOR).

Ingredients: 1 tablespoon dried flowers of viola tricolor, 250 ml boiling water.
Preparation: Infuse the flowers in boiling water for 10 minutes and strain.
Benefits: Promotes calmness and helps with evening agitation.
Suggested use: Drink one cup before bedtime.

15. CEDAR AND NEROLI ESSENTIAL OIL LOTION.

Ingredients: 2 drops cedar essential oil, 2 drops neroli essential oil, 1 tablespoon carrier oil.
Preparation: Mix the oils and apply with a massage to the wrists and solar plexus.
Benefits: Promotes a sense of serenity and makes it easier to fall asleep.
Usage tips: Use every evening.

16. FOOT BATH WITH SODIUM BICARBONATE AND LAVENDER.

Ingredients: 1 cup baking soda, 2 tablespoons dried lavender flowers, warm water.
Preparation: Mix baking soda and flowers in a bowl of warm water and soak feet for 15 minutes.
Benefits: Relaxes the body and calms the mind.
Usage tips: Make as needed, preferably before bedtime.

17. BERGAMOT AND ROMAN CHAMOMILE ESSENTIAL OIL LOTION.

Ingredients: 2 drops bergamot essential oil, 2 drops Roman chamomile essential oil, 1 tablespoon coconut oil.
Preparation: Mix oils and massage into temples and solar plexus.
Benefits: Promotes relaxation and reduces mild insomnia.
Usage tips: Apply as needed.

18. CALENDULA FLOWER INFUSION (CALENDULA OFFICINALIS).

Ingredients: 1 tablespoon dried calendula flowers, 250 ml boiling water.
Preparation: Infuse the flowers in boiling water for 10 minutes and strain.
Benefits: Soothes the nervous system and promotes peaceful sleep.
Usage tips: Drink one cup before bedtime.

19. HIMALAYAN PINK SALT AND MINT ESSENTIAL OIL BATH.

Ingredients: 2 cups of pink salt, 5 drops of mint essential oil, hot water.
Preparation: Dissolve the salt and oil in the hot water of the bath and soak for 20 minutes.
Benefits: Relaxes muscles and helps the mind relax.
Usage tips: Take the bath 1 time a week.

20. EUCALYPTUS AND LAVENDER ESSENTIAL OIL LOTION.

Ingredients: 2 drops eucalyptus essential oil, 2 drops lavender essential oil, 1 tablespoon carrier oil.
Preparation: Mix the oils and gently massage the feet and neck.
Benefits: Promotes relaxation and reduces physical tension before bedtime.
Usage tips: Apply every evening.

21. INFUSION OF HOP LEAVES (HUMULUS LUPULUS).

Ingredients: 1 teaspoon dried hop leaves, 250 ml boiling water.
Preparation: Pour boiling water over the leaves, let steep for 10 minutes and strain.

Benefits: Calming and sedative properties, ideal for mild insomnia.
Usage tips: Drink one cup before bedtime.

22. BASIL AND LAVENDER ESSENTIAL OIL LOTION.

Ingredients: 2 drops basil essential oil, 2 drops lavender essential oil, 1 tablespoon sweet almond oil.
Preparation: Mix the oils and gently massage the temples and nape of the neck.
Benefits: Reduces mental tension and promotes relaxation.
Usage tips: Apply every evening.

23. BATH WITH MAGNESIUM SALTS AND CHAMOMILE OIL.

Ingredients: 2 cups Epsom salts, 5 drops of chamomile essential oil, hot water.
Preparation: Dissolve the salts and oil in the hot water of the bath and soak for 20 minutes.
Benefits: Relieves muscle tension and promotes relaxing sleep.
Usage tips: Take the bath 1-2 times a week.

24. LEMON BALM AND VERBENA LEAVES HERBAL TEA.

Ingredients: 1 teaspoon dried lemon balm leaves, 1 teaspoon verbena, 250 ml boiling water.
Preparation: Infuse the herbs in boiling water for 10 minutes and strain.
Benefits: Calming and relaxing, helps prepare for sleep.
Usage tips: Drink one cup before bedtime.

25. TANGERINE AND ROMAN CHAMOMILE ESSENTIAL OIL LOTION.

Ingredients: 2 drops tangerine essential oil, 2 drops Roman chamomile essential oil, 1 tablespoon carrier oil.
Preparation: Mix the oils and massage the solar plexus and wrists.
Benefits: Promotes calm and reduces evening restlessness.
Usage tips: Use every evening.

26. FOOT BATH WITH LINDEN LEAVES AND EPSOM SALTS.

Ingredients: 1 tablespoon dried linden leaves, 1 cup Epsom salts, hot water.
Preparation: Mix the ingredients in a bowl of warm water and soak your feet for 15-20 minutes.
Benefits: Calms nerves and relaxes muscles.
Usage tips: Make as needed.

27. PATCHOULI AND SANDALWOOD ESSENTIAL OIL LOTION.

Ingredients: 2 drops patchouli essential oil, 2 drops sandalwood essential oil, 1 tablespoon coconut oil.
Preparation: Mix oils and gently massage feet and neck.
Benefits: Promotes deep grounding and relaxation.
Usage tips: Apply every evening.

28. GINGER ROOT AND LEMON INFUSION.

Ingredients: 1 teaspoon grated fresh ginger root, juice of half a lemon, 250 ml boiling water.
Preparation: Pour boiling water over ginger, add lemon and let steep for 10 minutes.
Benefits: Relaxes the body and facilitates evening relaxation.
Usage tips: Drink one cup before bedtime.

29. BATH WITH SEA SALT AND NEROLI OIL.

Ingredients: 2 cups of sea salt, 5 drops of neroli essential oil, hot water.
Preparation: Dissolve the salt and oil in the hot water in the bath and soak for 20 minutes.
Benefits: Relaxes muscles and promotes deep sleep.
Usage tips: Take the bath once a week.

30. GERANIUM AND LAVENDER ESSENTIAL OIL LOTION.

Ingredients: 2 drops geranium essential oil, 2 drops lavender essential oil, 1 tablespoon carrier oil.
Preparation: Mix the oils and massage into the solar plexus and wrists.
Benefits: Promotes relaxation and promotes restorative sleep.
Usage tips: Use every evening.

31. INFUSION OF PASSIONFLOWER AND HAWTHORN LEAVES.

Ingredients: 1 teaspoon dried passion flower leaves, 1 teaspoon hawthorn flowers, 250 ml boiling water.
Preparation: Infuse the herbs in boiling water for 10 minutes and strain.
Benefits: Reduces agitation and promotes deep sleep.
Usage tips: Drink one cup before bedtime.

32. VETIVER AND TANGERINE ESSENTIAL OIL LOTION.

Ingredients: 2 drops vetiver essential oil, 2 drops mandarin essential oil, 1 tablespoon coconut oil.
Preparation: Mix oils and gently massage temples and wrists.
Benefits: Promotes relaxation and a sense of deep calm.
Usage tips: Apply every evening.

33. BATH WITH GREEN CLAY AND ROSE OIL.

Ingredients: 1 cup green clay, 5 drops rose essential oil, warm water.
Preparation: Dissolve the clay and oil in the hot water in the bath and soak for 20 minutes.
Benefits: Purifies the skin and relaxes the muscles, promoting sleep.
Usage tips: Take the bath once a week.

34. FENNEL SEED AND PEPPERMINT HERBAL TEA.

Ingredients: 1 teaspoon fennel seeds, 1 teaspoon peppermint leaves, 250 ml boiling water.
Preparation: Infuse the seeds and leaves in boiling water for 10 minutes and strain.

Benefits: Soothes the stomach and relaxes the mind, promoting sleep.
Usage tips: Drink one cup after dinner.

35. YLANG YLANG AND HOLY BASIL ESSENTIAL OIL LOTION.

Ingredients: 2 drops ylang ylang essential oil, 2 drops sacred basil essential oil, 1 tablespoon carrier oil.
Preparation: Mix the oils and gently massage the neck and chest.
Benefits: Promotes muscle and mental relaxation.
Usage tips: Apply as needed.

36. FOOT BATH WITH ORANGE BLOSSOM WATER AND SEA SALT.

Ingredients: 2 tablespoons orange blossom water, 1 cup sea salt, hot water.
Preparation: Mix ingredients in a bowl of warm water and soak feet for 15 minutes.
Benefits: Relaxes the body and calms the nerves.
Usage tips: Make every night before bedtime.

37. CINNAMON AND NEROLI ESSENTIAL OIL LOTION.

Ingredients: 1 drop cinnamon essential oil, 2 drops neroli essential oil, 1 tablespoon sweet almond oil.
Preparation: Mix the oils and massage the solar plexus with gentle movements.
Benefits: Promotes calmness and reduces insomnia.
Usage tips: Apply every evening.

38. CALENDULA AND LIME BLOSSOM INFUSION.

Ingredients: 1 teaspoon marigold flowers, 1 teaspoon linden flowers, 250 ml boiling water.
Preparation: Infuse the flowers in boiling water for 10 minutes and strain.
Benefits: Soothes the nervous system and promotes peaceful sleep.
Usage tips: Drink one cup before bedtime.

39. BATH WITH EPSOM SALTS AND PATCHOULI ESSENTIAL OIL.

Ingredients: 2 cups Epsom salts, 5 drops patchouli essential oil, hot water.
Preparation: Dissolve the salts and oil in the hot water in the bath and soak for 20 minutes.
Benefits: Relaxes muscles and promotes deep sleep.
Usage tips: Take the bath once a week.

40. GERANIUM AND LEMONGRASS ESSENTIAL OIL LOTION.

Ingredients: 2 drops geranium essential oil, 2 drops lemongrass essential oil, 1 tablespoon carrier oil.
Preparation: Mix oils and gently massage temples and nape of neck.
Benefits: Promotes relaxation and relieves mental fatigue.
Usage tips: Apply every evening.

MENTAL ENERGY — NATURAL REMEDIES

Mental fatigue can affect concentration, memory and productivity. This section presents natural remedies to stimulate the mind, improve mental clarity and sustain energy levels without compromising well-being.

1. GINSENG (PANAX GINSENG) TINCTURE.

Ingredients: 1 tablespoon dried ginseng root, 100 ml edible alcohol (about 40°), 100 ml water.
Preparation: Mix alcohol and water in a jar, add the ginseng root and let macerate for 4 weeks in a dark place, shaking daily. Strain and store in a dark bottle.
Benefits: Natural stimulant, improves concentration and reduces mental fatigue.
Usage tips: Take 20 drops diluted in water in the morning or at the first sign of mental fatigue.

2. MATCHA GREEN TEA.

Ingredients: 1 teaspoon matcha powder, 250 ml hot water (not boiling, about 80°C).
Preparation: Pour the hot water over the matcha powder and stir vigorously with a bamboo whisk until it forms a light foam.
Benefits: Rich in antioxidants and L-theanine, it improves concentration and provides stable energy without jitters.
Usage tips: Drink one cup in the morning or during an energy slump.

3. YERBA MATE (ILEX PARAGUARIENSIS) INFUSION.

Ingredients: 1 tablespoon dried yerba mate leaves, 250 ml hot water (about 80°C).
Preparation: Pour hot water over the leaves and let infuse for 5-7 minutes. Strain.
Benefits: Natural energizer, improves mental alertness and mood.
Usage tips: Drink one cup as needed, avoiding evening consumption.

4. ROSEMARY AND MINT ESSENTIAL OIL LOTION.

Ingredients: 2 drops rosemary essential oil, 2 drops peppermint essential oil, 1 tablespoon sweet almond oil.
Preparation: Mix the oils and gently massage the temples and nape of the neck.
Benefits: Stimulates the mind and promotes mental clarity.
Usage tips: Apply as needed during times of mental fatigue.

5. ELEUTHEROCOCCUS ROOT (ELEUTHEROCOCCUS SENTICOSUS) DECOCTION.

Ingredients: 1 teaspoon dried eleutherococcus root, 300 ml water.
Preparation: Bring water with the root to a boil, simmer for 10 minutes and strain.
Benefits: Adaptogen that improves stress resistance and supports mental energy levels.
Usage tips: Drink one cup in the morning.

6. GINKGO BILOBA LEAF HERBAL TEA.

Ingredients: 1 teaspoon dried ginkgo biloba leaves, 250 ml boiling water.
Preparation: Pour boiling water over the leaves and let steep for 10 minutes. Strain.

Benefits: Improves cerebral circulation, promoting memory and concentration.
Usage tips: Drink one cup in the morning or afternoon.

7. LEMON AND ROSEMARY ESSENTIAL OIL LOTION.

Ingredients: 2 drops lemon essential oil, 2 drops rosemary essential oil, 1 tablespoon jojoba oil.
Preparation: Mix the oils and apply with gentle massage to the temples and nape of the neck.
Benefits: Energizing and stimulating, helps fight mental fatigue.
Usage tips: Use as needed.

8. MATCHA AND SPINACH SMOOTHIE.

Ingredients: 1 teaspoon matcha powder, 1 handful fresh spinach, 1 banana, 250 ml vegetable milk (almond or coconut).
Preparation: Blend all ingredients until smooth.
Benefits: Provides stable energy and promotes concentration due to the combination of matcha and spinach nutrients.
Usage tips: Consume in the morning or as an afternoon snack.

9. LEMON MINT ESSENTIAL OIL LOTION.

Ingredients: 2 drops peppermint essential oil, 2 drops lemon essential oil, 1 tablespoon carrier oil.
Preparation: Mix oils and gently massage wrists and neck.
Benefits: Stimulates the mind and improves alertness.
Usage tips: Apply as needed throughout the day.

10. MACA ROOT (LEPIDIUM MEYENII) INFUSION.

Ingredients: 1 teaspoon maca root powder, 250 ml hot (not boiling) water.
Preparation: Stir the powder into the hot water until completely dissolved.
Benefits: Natural energizer, improves mental and physical stamina.
Usage tips: Drink one cup in the morning.

11. ASTRAGALUS ROOT (ASTRAGALUS MEMBRANACEUS) INFUSION.

Ingredients: 1 teaspoon dried astragalus root, 250 ml boiling water.
Preparation: Pour boiling water over the root, let steep for 10 minutes and strain.
Benefits: Adaptogen that helps fight mental fatigue and improves stress resistance.
Usage tips: Drink one cup in the morning.

12. EUCALYPTUS AND PEPPERMINT ESSENTIAL OIL LOTION.

Ingredients: 2 drops eucalyptus essential oil, 2 drops peppermint essential oil, 1 tablespoon carrier oil.
Preparation: Mix the oils and gently massage the temples and nape of the neck.
Benefits: Invigorating and stimulating, promotes mental clarity.
Usage tips: Apply as needed.

13. SMOOTHIE WITH GUARANA AND BERRIES.

Ingredients: 1 teaspoon guarana powder, 1 handful fresh berries, 1 banana, 250 ml vegetable milk.
Preparation: Blend all ingredients until creamy consistency.
Benefits: Boosts mental and physical energy thanks to guarana and the antioxidants in berries.
Usage tips: Consume in the morning or as an afternoon snack.

14. DANDELION ROOT DECOCTION (TARAXACUM OFFICINALE).

Ingredients: 1 teaspoon dried dandelion root, 300 ml water.
Preparation: Bring water with the root to a boil, simmer for 10 minutes and strain.
Benefits: Purifying and invigorating, helps improve energy levels.
Usage tips: Drink one cup in the morning.

15. LEMONGRASS AND HOLY BASIL ESSENTIAL OIL LOTION.

Ingredients: 2 drops lemongrass essential oil, 2 drops holy basil essential oil, 1 tablespoon coconut oil.
Preparation: Mix the oils and massage the neck and wrists.
Benefits: Stimulates the mind and relieves mental fatigue.
Usage tips: Use as needed.

16. ROSEMARY AND SAGE HERBAL TEA.

Ingredients: 1 teaspoon dried rosemary leaves, 1 teaspoon sage leaves, 250 ml boiling water.
Preparation: Infuse the herbs in boiling water for 10 minutes and strain.
Benefits: Improves memory and promotes concentration.
Usage tips: Drink one cup in the morning.

17. SCOTS PINE AND MINT ESSENTIAL OIL LOTION.

Ingredients: 2 drops Scots pine essential oil, 2 drops peppermint essential oil, 1 tablespoon carrier oil.
Preparation: Mix the oils and massage the solar plexus and temples.
Benefits: Promotes mental clarity and reduces feelings of fatigue.
Usage tips: Apply as needed.

18. INFUSION OF SCHISANDRA BERRY (SCHISANDRA CHINENSIS).

Ingredients: 1 teaspoon dried schisandra berries, 250 ml boiling water.
Preparation: Pour boiling water over the berries, let steep for 10 minutes and strain.
Benefits: Adaptogen that improves concentration and reduces mental stress.
Usage tips: Drink one cup in the morning.

19. BERGAMOT AND YLANG YLANG ESSENTIAL OIL LOTION.

Ingredients: 2 drops bergamot essential oil, 2 drops ylang ylang essential oil, 1 tablespoon sweet almond oil.
Preparation: Mix the oils and apply with gentle massage to the temples and neck.

Benefits: Refreshing and balancing, promotes mental energy.
Usage tips: Use as needed.

20. BURDOCK ROOT (ARCTIUM LAPPA) DECOCTION.

Ingredients: 1 teaspoon dried burdock root, 300 ml water.
Preparation: Bring water with root to a boil, simmer for 10 minutes and strain.
Benefits: Purifying and invigorating, ideal for improving mental energy levels.
Usage tips: Drink one cup in the morning.

21. GOJI BERRY AND GINGER HERBAL TEA.

Ingredients: 1 tablespoon goji berries, 1 teaspoon grated fresh ginger, 250 ml boiling water.
Preparation: Infuse the berries and ginger in boiling water for 10 minutes and strain.
Benefits: Provides antioxidants and improves mental vitality.
Usage tips: Drink one cup in the morning.

22. SWEET ORANGE AND ROSEMARY ESSENTIAL OIL LOTION.

Ingredients: 2 drops sweet orange essential oil, 2 drops rosemary essential oil, 1 tablespoon carrier oil.
Preparation: Mix the oils and gently massage the wrists and temples.
Benefits: Stimulates concentration and reduces mental fatigue.
Usage tips: Apply during dips in energy.

23. ELDERFLOWER AND LEMON INFUSION.

Ingredients: 1 teaspoon dried elderflowers, juice of half a lemon, 250 ml boiling water.
Preparation: Pour boiling water over flowers, add lemon and let steep for 10 minutes. Strain.
Benefits: Refreshing and invigorating, promotes mental clarity.
Usage tips: Drink one cup in the morning or afternoon.

24. CYPRESS LEMON ESSENTIAL OIL LOTION.

Ingredients: 2 drops cypress essential oil, 2 drops lemon essential oil, 1 tablespoon jojoba oil.
Preparation: Mix the oils and massage into temples and solar plexus.
Benefits: Promotes mental clarity and reduces feelings of fatigue.
Usage tips: Use as needed.

25. SMOOTHIE WITH SPIRULINA AND BANANA

Ingredients: 1 teaspoon spirulina powder, 1 banana, 250 ml vegetable milk (soy or almond).
Preparation: Blend all ingredients until smooth.
Benefits: Spirulina provides essential nutrients and improves mental energy levels.
Usage tips: Consume in the morning or as an afternoon snack.

26. HOLY BASIL (TULSI) AND PEPPERMINT LEAVES HERBAL TEA.

Ingredients: 1 teaspoon dried holy basil leaves, 1 teaspoon peppermint leaves, 250 ml boiling water.
Preparation: Infuse herbs in boiling water for 10 minutes and strain.
Benefits: Improves concentration and helps relax the mind.
Usage tips: Drink one cup in the morning.

27. NEROLI AND SAGE ESSENTIAL OIL LOTION.

Ingredients: 2 drops neroli essential oil, 2 drops sage essential oil, 1 tablespoon sweet almond oil.
Preparation: Mix the oils and gently massage the temples and nape of the neck.
Benefits: Helps restore mental energy and reduces stress.
Usage tips: Use as needed.

28. LICORICE ROOT AND GINGER DECOCTION.

Ingredients: 1 teaspoon licorice root, 1 teaspoon grated fresh ginger, 300 ml water.
Preparation: Bring water with ingredients to a boil, simmer for 10 minutes and strain.
Benefits: Energizing and stimulating, useful for a tired mind.
Usage tips: Drink one cup in the morning.

29. WINTERGREEN AND ROSEMARY ESSENTIAL OIL LOTION.

Ingredients: 2 drops wintergreen essential oil, 2 drops rosemary essential oil, 1 tablespoon coconut oil.
Preparation: Mix oils and massage solar plexus and wrists.
Benefits: Promotes concentration and reduces mental fatigue.
Usage tips: Apply throughout the day.

30. CHIA SEED AND LEMON INFUSION.

Ingredients: 1 tablespoon chia seeds, juice of half a lemon, 250 ml hot water.
Preparation: Mix ingredients and let stand for 10 minutes.
Benefits: Provides stable energy and helps improve concentration.
Usage tips: Drink in the morning or during an energy slump.

31. ROSEMARY AND LEMON HERBAL TEA.

Ingredients: 1 teaspoon dried rosemary leaves, zest of half a lemon, 250 ml boiling water.
Preparation: Pour boiling water over ingredients, let steep for 10 minutes and strain.
Benefits: Natural tonic for the mind, helps improve concentration.
Usage tips: Drink one cup in the morning or afternoon.

32. THYME AND LEMON ESSENTIAL OIL LOTION.

Ingredients: 2 drops thyme essential oil, 2 drops lemon essential oil, 1 tablespoon carrier oil.
Preparation: Mix the oils and gently massage the neck and temples.

Benefits: Energizing and stimulating, reduces mental fatigue.
Usage tips: Use as needed.

33. INFUSION OF MINT LEAVES AND CALENDULA FLOWERS.

Ingredients: 1 teaspoon mint leaves, 1 teaspoon dried calendula flowers, 250 ml boiling water.
Preparation: Infuse ingredients in boiling water for 10 minutes and strain.
Benefits: Refreshing and calming, promotes mental clarity.
Usage tips: Drink one cup during a drop in energy.

34. LAVENDER AND CYPRESS ESSENTIAL OIL LOTION.

Ingredients: 2 drops lavender essential oil, 2 drops cypress essential oil, 1 tablespoon sweet almond oil.
Preparation: Mix oils and massage wrists and neck.
Benefits: Promotes relaxation and concentration.
Usage tips: Apply during times of mental fatigue.

35. SMOOTHIE WITH AVOCADO AND MATCHA.

Ingredients: 1/2 ripe avocado, 1 teaspoon matcha powder, 1 tablespoon honey, 250 ml vegetable milk.
Preparation: Blend all ingredients to a creamy consistency.
Benefits: Energizing and nourishing, ideal for supporting the mind during busy days.
Usage tips: Consume in the morning or afternoon.

36. BURDOCK ROOT AND LEMON HERBAL TEA.

Ingredients: 1 teaspoon dried burdock root, juice of half a lemon, 250 ml boiling water.
Preparation: Infuse the root in boiling water for 10 minutes, then add lemon juice and strain.
Benefits: Purifying and stimulating for the mind.
Usage tips: Drink one cup in the morning.

37. GERANIUM AND ROSEMARY ESSENTIAL OIL LOTION.

Ingredients: 2 drops geranium essential oil, 2 drops rosemary essential oil, 1 tablespoon carrier oil.
Preparation: Mix oils and massage into temples and solar plexus.
Benefits: Stimulates mental energy and improves alertness.
Usage tips: Use as needed.

38. LAVENDER AND ROSEMARY FLOWER INFUSION.

Ingredients: 1 teaspoon lavender flowers, 1 teaspoon rosemary leaves, 250 ml boiling water.
Preparation: Pour boiling water over ingredients, let steep for 10 minutes and strain.
Benefits: Calms nerves and promotes concentration.
Usage tips: Drink one cup in the afternoon.

39. BERGAMOT AND SAGE ESSENTIAL OIL LOTION.

Ingredients: 2 drops bergamot essential oil, 2 drops sage essential oil, 1 tablespoon coconut oil.
Preparation: Mix the oils and massage into the neck and wrists.
Benefits: Promotes mental relaxation and clarity.
Usage tips: Apply as needed.

40. ELEUTHEROCOCCUS ROOT AND LICORICE DECOCTION.

Ingredients: 1 teaspoon eleutherococcus root, 1 teaspoon licorice root, 300 ml water.
Preparation: Bring ingredients to a boil with water, simmer for 10 minutes and strain.
Benefits: Stimulates the mind and fights mental fatigue.
Usage tips: Drink one cup in the morning.

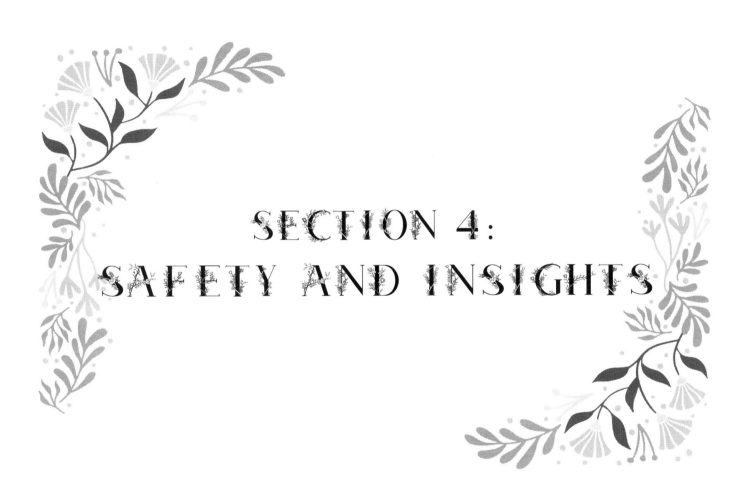

SECTION 4:
SAFETY AND INSIGHTS

CHAPTER 10:
SAFETY AND DOSAGES

Home pharmacy is a powerful tool for promoting wellness, but like any health-related practice, it requires responsibility and awareness. Herbs, despite their natural origin, possess active ingredients that can interact with our bodies in complex ways. Safety in the use of medicinal plants is a matter of balance: recognizing the benefits without neglecting the potential risks.

In this chapter we will explore the basic guidelines for safe and effective use of herbal remedies. You will learn how to calculate dosages, understand drug interactions, and identify situations where the use of specific herbs may be contraindicated. This will enable you to use your home pharmacy with confidence, respecting the limits of each remedy and promoting responsible herbal practice.

Get ready to build the foundation for a safe and conscious approach to natural health, guided by simple and clear rules that protect you and your loved ones.

RECOMMENDED DOSAGES

TABLES FOR TINCTURES, HERBAL TEAS AND OILS

One of the most critical aspects in the preparation and use of herbal remedies is dosage. Proper dosage maximizes therapeutic benefits and minimizes risks. Although herbal remedies are generally safe when used appropriately, excessive or incorrect doses can lead to unwanted side effects or, in extreme cases, toxicity.

This section provides detailed tables to help you accurately dose tinctures, herbal teas, and oils. However, it is always advisable to start with low doses, carefully observe how the body responds, and gradually increase if necessary.

1. TINCTURES: GENERAL DOSAGES

Tinctures are extracted liquid concentrates and require special attention in dosing. Here is a table with guidelines for the most common tinctures:

Herb	Primary Use	Recommended Daily Dosage	Important Notes
Echinacea	Immune Support	20-30 drops, 2-3 times a day	Do not use continuously for more than 2 weeks.
Valerian	Anxiety, Insomnia	15-20 drops, before bedtime	May cause drowsiness; avoid driving.
Hawthorn	Heart Health	15-25 drops, 3 times a day	Do not combine with heart medications without medical advice.
Devil's Claw	Joint Pain	20 drops, 2 times a day	Avoid in cases of gastric ulcers.
Chamomile	Digestion, Relaxation	15-20 drops, 3 times a day	Safe for children in reduced doses.

2. HERBAL TEAS AND INFUSIONS: GENERAL DOSAGES

Herbal teas are one of the easiest and safest ways to take medicinal herbs. The following table shows the recommended dosages for preparation:

Herb	Primary Use	Amount per Cup (250 ml)	Recommended Daily Dosage
Chamomile	Relaxation, Digestion	1 teaspoon of dried flowers	Up to 3 cups per day.
Mint	Digestion, Nausea	1-2 teaspoons of dried leaves	Up to 3 cups per day.
Ginger	Nausea, Inflammation	1 teaspoon of freshly grated root	2-3 cups per day.
Linden	Relaxation, Fever	1 teaspoon of dried flowers	1-2 cups per day.
Mallow	Cough, Sore Throat	2 teaspoons of dried flowers	1-3 cups per day.

3. ESSENTIAL OILS AND INFUSIONS: USE AND DOSAGES

Essential oils are potent and should be used with extreme caution. Infused oils, on the other hand, are safer and suitable for daily use.

Type of Oil	Primary Use	Recommended Dosage	Important Notes
Lavender Oil	Relaxation, Irritated Skin	2-3 drops in a diffuser or carrier oil	Do not apply directly to the skin.
Mint Oil	Headache, Nausea	1 drop in carrier oil, applied to temples	Avoid contact with eyes.
Calendula Oil	Hydration, Minor Wounds	Apply pure or diluted to small areas	Also suitable for children.
St. John's Wort Oil	Sunburn, Muscle Pain	Apply 1-2 times per day	Avoid sun exposure after application.
Tea Tree Oil	Antibacterial, Acne	1 drop in 10 ml of carrier oil	Do not ingest; for topical use only

GENERAL DOSING TIPS

- Start with minimum doses: Always evaluate the body's reaction.
- Stick to daily limits: Do not exceed the recommended amounts.
- Consult an expert: If you have medical conditions or are taking medications, seek advice from a herbalist or doctor.
- Always dilute essential oils: They are extremely concentrated and can cause irritation if used pure.

THE 10 GOLDEN RULES FOR SAFE DOSING.

1. Read the directions for each remedy carefully.
2. Use accurate measuring tools (pipettes, scales).
3. Do not experiment with unfamiliar herbs without reliable information.
4. Avoid high doses for prolonged periods.
5. Keep a diary to monitor effects and progress.
6. Do not combine remedies without specific knowledge.
7. Avoid using herbs in pregnancy without supervision.
8. Store preparations in safe places, out of the reach of children.
9. Discontinue use immediately in case of adverse reactions.
10. Be patient: natural remedies act gradually.

INTERACTIONS WITH MEDICATIONS

WHAT TO AVOID

One of the most sensitive aspects of using medicinal herbs is their interaction with conventional medications. Plants contain natural chemical compounds that can enhance, reduce or alter the effect of some medicines, sometimes with serious consequences. It is essential to know about these interactions in order to use herbal remedies safely and responsibly.

1. THE MOST COMMON HERBS AND THEIR INTERACTIONS.

Here is a list of the most commonly used herbs and known interactions with conventional drugs:

Herb	Medications It Interacts With	Effects of Interaction	Important Notes
St. John's Wort	Antidepressants, oral contraceptives	Reduces the effectiveness of contraceptives and alters mood	Avoid with SSRIs or MAO inhibitors.
Ginseng	Anticoagulants, heart medications	May increase the risk of bleeding	Avoid with warfarin or aspirin.
Licorice	Blood pressure medications	May raise blood pressure	Avoid with blood pressure medications.
Valerian	Sedatives, antidepressants	May enhance sedation	Avoid with benzodiazepines or alcohol.
Garlic	Anticoagulants	Increases the risk of bleeding	Avoid with drugs like warfarin.
Ginkgo Biloba	Anticoagulants, antiepileptic drugs	May increase the risk of bleeding or reduce drug effectiveness	Consult a doctor.
Chamomile	Anticoagulants, sedatives	May enhance sedative or blood-thinning effects	Avoid high doses with specific medications.
Echinacea	Immunosuppressants	May reduce the effectiveness of medications for transplants or autoimmune conditions	Short-term use recommended.

2. CLASSIFICATION OF INTERACTIONS

Herb-drug interactions can be classified into three main categories:
1. **Potentiating Interactions:**
   o Some herbs can amplify the effects of drugs, increasing the risk of toxicity.
   o Example: Valerian increases the effect of sedatives, causing extreme drowsiness.

2. **Antagonistic Interactions:**
   o Other herbs can reduce the effectiveness of drugs by interfering with their absorption or metabolism.
   o Example: St. John's Wort reduces the effectiveness of oral contraceptives.

3. **Indirect Interactions:**
   o Some herbs affect hepatic metabolism through enzymes such as cytochrome P450, changing the rate at which drugs are metabolized.
   o Example: Ginseng can accelerate the metabolism of some drugs, reducing their duration of action.

3. RISK GROUPS.

Some people are particularly vulnerable to herb-drug interactions. In these cases, it is essential to consult a doctor or qualified herbalist:
- **Pregnant or lactating women**: Avoid potent herbs such as St. John's Wort, mugwort or licorice.
- **Older people**: They are more susceptible to side effects and interactions.
- **Children**: They have less developed metabolic systems; even small doses must be adjusted carefully.
- **Patients with chronic diseases**: Such as diabetes, heart, liver or kidney disease.

4. HOW TO PREVENT INTERACTIONS

To use herbal remedies safely, follow these guidelines:
1. **Consult a professional**: Before introducing new herbs into your routine, inform your doctor or pharmacist, especially if you take prescribed medications.
2. **Avoid do-it-yourself in complex cases**: Do not take herbal remedies in serious situations or when you are unsure of interactions.
3. **Start with one herb at a time**: This way, you can monitor your body's reactions.
4. **Avoid high doses**: Interactions are more likely with concentrated doses, such as tinctures or high-potency capsules.
5. **Monitor symptoms**: If you notice side effects, discontinue use and consult an expert.

HERBS TO USE WITH GREATER CAUTION.

Here is a list of herbs that require special attention for their powerful properties:
- **Hypericum**: Powerful enzyme inducer, interacts with numerous drugs.
- **Garlic**: Blood thinner; caution during surgery.
- **Ginseng**: May alter blood sugar; caution in diabetics.
- **Ginkgo biloba**: Increases risk of bleeding, especially with anticoagulants.
- **Valerian**: Potentiates sedatives and alcohol.

AT-RISK GROUPS

PREGNANCY, LACTATION AND CHILDREN

Certain groups of people, such as pregnant or lactating women and children, are particularly sensitive to the effects of medicinal herbs. In these cases, the use of natural remedies requires an extremely cautious approach. Even plants considered safe may have unforeseen effects due to biological changes, high dosages, or interactions with the ongoing development of the fetus or child.

1. HERBS AND PREGNANCY

During pregnancy, the female body undergoes significant changes that can alter the way herbs are metabolized. Some plants can stimulate uterine contractions, alter hormones, or interfere with fetal development.

HERBS TO AVOID IN PREGNANCY

Herb	Reason for Risk	Potential Effects
Mugwort (Artemisia)	Stimulates uterine contractions	Risk of miscarriage.
Sage (Salvia officinalis)	Contains thujone, a neurotoxic substance	Risk to the fetal nervous system.
Ginseng	May alter hormone levels	Risk of abnormalities in fetal development.
St. John's Wort	Interferes with hormone levels	Potential interference in fetal development.
Aloe Vera (internal use)	Powerful laxative, stimulates uterine contractions	Risk to pregnancy.

SAFE HERBS FOR PREGNANCY

Not all herbs are to be avoided. Some plants can be helpful in managing common pregnancy symptoms such as nausea, insomnia, or difficult digestion.

Herb	Primary Use	Usage Method
Ginger	Reduces nausea and vomiting	Infusion or small doses of fresh root.
Chamomile	Relaxes and aids sleep	Light tea, 1-2 cups per day.
Mallow	Helps with constipation and inflammation	Infusion for digestive issues.
Linden	Relaxation, cardiovascular support	Herbal tea to relieve stress.

2. HERBS AND LACTATION

Substances in herbs can be transferred to the infant through breast milk. It is essential to use only plants that are considered safe for the baby.

HERBS TO AVOID WHILE BREASTFEEDING

Herb	Reason for Risk	Potential Effects
Peppermint	May reduce milk production	Risk of insufficient milk supply.
Sage (Salvia officinalis)	Inhibits lactation	Significant reduction in breast milk.
St. John's Wort	May alter the newborn's mood	Possible sleep disturbances.

SAFE HERBS DURING BREASTFEEDING

Herb	Primary Use	Usage Method
Fennel	Stimulates milk production	Infusion or seeds added to meals
Nettle	Supports milk production	Infusion, rich in nutrients like iron and calcium
Chamomile	Calming for mother and baby	Light tea, promotes relaxation

3. HERBS AND CHILDREN

Children are particularly sensitive to the effects of herbs because of their low body weight and developing immune systems. Remedies must be tailored to their needs with low dosages and extreme care.

HERBS TO AVOID IN CHILDREN

Herb	Reason for Risk	Potential Effects
Peppermint Essential Oil	May cause respiratory spasms in infants	Dangerous even in small amounts.
Ginseng	Overly stimulating for the nervous system	Risk of hyperactivity or insomnia.
Mugwort (Artemisia)	Potential toxicity	Neurotoxic effects.

SAFE HERBS FOR CHILDREN

Herb	Primary Use	Usage Method
Chamomile	Calming, reduces colic	Light infusion, 1 teaspoon of dried flowers.
Mallow	Cough, throat irritation	Herbal tea or gargles (for older children).
Lemon Balm	Helps with anxiety and restlessness	Light infusion, 1 cup divided into 2 doses.

4. GENERAL GUIDELINES FOR RISK GROUPS.

Consult an expert: Before using herbs when pregnant, breastfeeding or with children, always seek advice from a qualified physician or herbalist.

- **Avoid DIY**: Do not use potent herbs without extensive knowledge.
- **Use minimal doses**: Adjust the dosage according to the recipient's body weight and sensitivity.
- **Watch reactions carefully**: Discontinue use immediately if side effects occur.
- **Store preparations safely**: Away from the reach of young children to avoid accidental ingestion.

PRACTICAL BOX: THE 5 FAMILY FRIENDLY HERBS.

1. Chamomile: Versatile and safe for moms and children.
2. Mallow: Perfect for coughs and inflammation.
3. Lemon Balm: Ideal for anxiety and irritability.
4. Fennel: A natural aid for digestion and milk production.
5. Linden: Relaxing for the whole family.

CHAPTER 11:
TIPS FOR GROWING MEDICINAL HERBS IN YOUR GARDEN OR BALCONY

CHOOSING THE RIGHT HERBS - COMPATIBILITY WITH CLIMATE AND SPACE

Growing medicinal herbs in one's garden or balcony is a practice that combines the fascination of nature with the satisfaction of creating home remedies with plants grown with one's own hands. However, successful cultivation depends on choosing the right herbs, which must be compatible with the local climate and available space. This initial stage is crucial to ensure healthy and productive plants.

First, it is important to consider the climate of your area. Each plant has specific needs for temperature, sun exposure and humidity. For example, if you live in an area with hot, dry summers, Mediterranean herbs such as rosemary, sage and thyme are good choices, as they thrive in dry, sunny conditions. In contrast, in cooler or wetter climates, plants such as mint, parsley and valerian may be better adapted, due to their tolerance of milder temperatures and higher soil moisture.

In addition to climate, available space plays an essential role in choosing herbs. If you have a large garden, you can opt for plants that expand easily, such as lavender or St. John's Wort, creating a lush, fragrant corner. However, if you are working with limited space, such as a balcony or windowsill, compact herbs such as basil, lemon balm and chamomile are more suitable. These plants can be grown in pots and require less root space while still maintaining a generous yield.

Another factor to consider is sun exposure. Medicinal herbs are generally sun-loving plants, but not all tolerate the same intensity. A south-facing balcony may be perfect for thyme and oregano, which love direct light for many hours a day. On the other hand, if your space receives only partial light or shade, herbs such as nettle and bear garlic, which prefer cooler, shaded environments, may be an ideal option.

The type of soil or substrate you will use should not be forgotten. In the garden, it is important to know the natural composition of the soil and, if necessary, enrich it with organic compost to improve fertility. For pots, a light, well-drained mixture is the best choice. Herbs such as marigold and dandelion require richer soil, while plants such as sage and rosemary prefer poorer, well-drained soils.

Finally, your choice of herbs should be in line with your main purpose. If you intend to make relaxing herbal teas, herbs such as lemon balm and linden are ideal. If, on the other hand, you want skin remedies, opt for calendula or plantain. Growing plants that you use frequently in your home pharmacy ensures not only personal satisfaction, but also more practical and immediate use of your crops.

In summary, choosing the right herbs for your garden or balcony means finding the right balance between climate, space and personal needs. It is a process that requires observation and planning, but in return offers a deep connection with nature and the joy of growing plants that can turn into valuable remedies for your health.

CULTIVATION TECHNIQUES - SOIL, IRRIGATION, SUN EXPOSURE

Growing medicinal herbs requires attention and care to meet the specific needs of each plant. Soil, irrigation and sun exposure are the pillars on which to build healthy, lush growth. With a conscious approach, even the simplest spaces can be transformed into little green havens, full of useful herbs for your home pharmacy.

Soil is the first element to consider. Medicinal herbs grow best in a well-drained, fertile substrate that allows roots to breathe and absorb nutrients. For garden growers, a light, friable soil is ideal, but it can be improved by adding organic compost or sand to increase porosity. In pots, on the other hand, it is essential to use herb-specific potting soil or create a custom mixture. A good base is two parts all-purpose potting soil, one part sand and one part compost. This combination provides the necessary drainage and a balanced supply of nutrients. It is important to avoid soils that are too rich in clay, which retains water, or too sandy, which disperses it quickly.

Irrigation is equally crucial and requires a balanced approach. Most medicinal herbs do not like stagnant water, which can cause root rot and weaken the plant. However, it is equally important to prevent the soil from drying out completely, especially during the germination phase or during warmer periods. Ideal watering depends on the type of grass and the climate. Plants such as rosemary and sage, which come from Mediterranean environments, require moderate watering, letting the soil dry out between watering. In contrast, herbs such as mint or parsley, which prefer wetter environments, require more frequent watering. Water should be given directly at the base of the plant, avoiding overwatering the leaves, which can develop fungal diseases if they remain moist for too long.

Sun exposure is a key determinant of photosynthesis and, consequently, of herb health and productivity. Most medicinal herbs prefer a sunny location, with at least six hours of direct light per day. However, not all plants have the same requirements. Mediterranean herbs such as thyme, oregano and lavender thrive in full sun and warm conditions. On the other hand, plants such as nettle, valerian and bear garlic prefer partial exposure or bright shade, as they naturally grow in wooded areas or along shady edges. When growing on a balcony, it is helpful to carefully observe how the sun moves during the day to choose the best locations for each plant.

An additional consideration concerns the microclimate. For example, a garden exposed to wind will require protections such as hedges or barriers, while a balcony in full sun might benefit from shade curtains during the hottest hours to avoid stressing the plants. In pots, drainage becomes even more important: saucers should never hold stagnant water, and the bottom of the pot should have holes in it to encourage the removal of excess moisture.

In summary, growing medicinal herbs requires constant attention to soil characteristics, irrigation and sun exposure. Learning to observe plant needs and respond to environmental conditions is one of the keys to a lush and satisfying harvest. With a little practice, any green space, large or small, can be transformed into a haven for healthy herbs ready to be used in your home remedies.

VERTICAL GARDENS AND CONTAINERS - SOLUTIONS FOR SMALL SPACES

Even with limited space, growing medicinal herbs can become a reality with creative solutions such as vertical gardens and the use of containers. These methods not only maximize space utilization but also add a decorative green touch to your environment, transforming balconies, terraces, and even interior walls into oases of wellness.

The vertical garden is one of the most versatile techniques for those who live in apartments or have a small balcony. The idea is simple: grow plants vertically instead of horizontally, taking advantage of structures such as grids, pallets, or pocket panels. Fabric pockets are particularly useful because they hold soil but allow water to drain freely, preventing stagnation that could damage roots. Alternatively, you can use multi-level shelving with pots arranged on each shelf, ensuring that each plant receives sufficient light. This approach works well for herbs such as mint, chamomile and lemon balm, which do not require particularly deep roots.

For those who prefer a simpler solution, individual containers are a practical and flexible option. Pots can be hung from railings, attached to walls, or arranged on shelves along the balcony. The choice of containers is important: lightweight materials such as recycled plastic or breathable fabrics are ideal to make it easier to move the pots and to prevent roots from overheating in the summer months. To maximize space, cascading pots can be used, where several containers are stacked in a pyramid structure, allowing several plants to be grown in one spot.

One of the advantages of containers is the ability to customize the soil and irrigation for each individual plant. For example, you can grow Mediterranean plants such as rosemary and thyme in pots with well-drained, sandier soil, while herbs such as parsley and mint can thrive in wetter, nutrient-rich potting soils. This flexibility allows you to grow a variety of herbs even in small spaces, without compromising on their health.

A key aspect to consider in vertical and container gardens is irrigation. In a compact environment, plants can dry out more quickly than those grown in the ground. For ease of maintenance, you can install a drip irrigation system, which is especially useful for green walls or crowded balconies. These systems distribute water evenly and gradually, reducing waste and ensuring that each plant gets the hydration it needs.

Another practical tip for maximizing space is to take advantage of multipurpose supports such as old wooden ladders, fruit crates, or climbing racks. These items can be easily transformed into structures to hold pots or to grow climbing herbs such as hops or borage. Not only do they save space, but they also lend a rustic, natural look to your green space.

Finally, for those without access to a balcony or garden, even a windowsill can become an ideal place to grow herbs in small pots. In these cases, the use of containers with self-watering systems is particularly beneficial, as it reduces the need for frequent watering and ensures constant moisture for the roots.

In conclusion, whether you have a large space or just a small corner, vertical gardens and containers offer endless possibilities for growing medicinal herbs. With a little creativity and planning, you can turn even the most modest of spaces into a green pharmacy, ready to provide fresh, healthy ingredients for your home remedies.

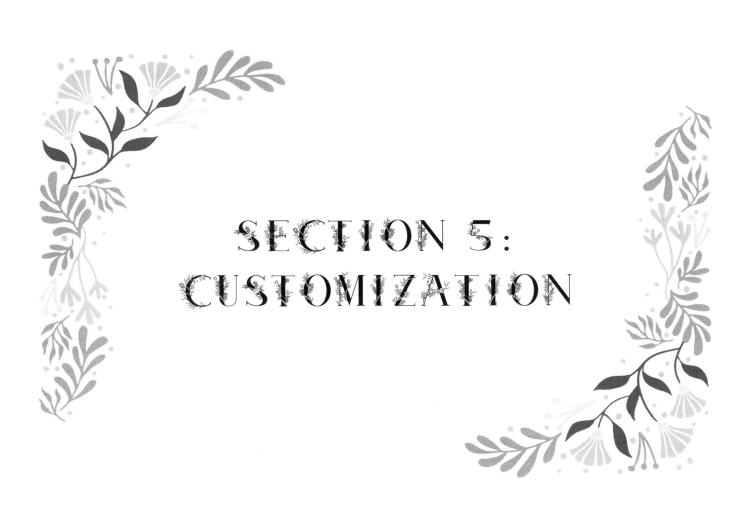

SECTION 5: CUSTOMIZATION

CHAPTER 12:
CREATING RECIPES TAILORED FOR EVERY NEED

WHY CUSTOMIZE REMEDIES?

Personalization of herbal remedies represents a unique and intimate journey to wellness. Every individual is different, with needs, preferences, and conditions that deserve specific attention. Creating personalized remedies is not only a way to tailor preparations to one's needs, but also an opportunity to deepen one's connection with nature and oneself.

To customize is to be in control. In a world where many products are standardized and often designed for an indistinct mass of consumers, herbal remedies offer a valuable alternative: you can choose what works best for you. For example, a relaxing herbal tea might have a powerful effect on one person but be too mild or even ineffective for another. By adjusting the proportions of the herbs, introducing a spice to enhance the aroma or a natural sweetener to make it more palatable, you transform a simple drink into a unique blend, calibrated to your needs.

Then there is the aspect of tolerability. Every body reacts differently to natural ingredients. Customizing allows one to avoid plants that may not be well tolerated or even cause unwanted reactions, choosing safe and equally effective alternatives. This process allows you to respect your sensitivities without sacrificing the benefits of herbalism.

In addition to meeting physical needs, customization also has strong emotional value. It creates a special bond between those who prepare the remedy and those who use it. Each recipe becomes an experience, an opportunity to explore new flavors, scents and textures that can evoke memories, comfort the soul or simply improve the mood. It is an invitation to creativity, experimentation and self-discovery.

Finally, personalizing is a form of empathy and healing. Preparing a specific remedy for a family member or friend, carefully choosing herbs based on their preferences and needs, is a gesture that communicates care and love. This practice goes beyond simple technical preparation-it becomes a ritual of sharing and connection.

Personalizing herbal remedies, then, is not just a matter of efficiency or preference, but a comprehensive approach to wellness that integrates body, mind, and spirit in a single act of care.

ADAPTING RECIPES TO INDIVIDUAL NEEDS: TASTES, HEALTH CONDITIONS, AVAILABILITY OF INGREDIENTS

Tailoring recipes to individual needs is a key step in creating effective and enjoyable herbal remedies. Each person has taste preferences, specific health conditions, and varying availability of ingredients, and these variables influence how a remedy is prepared and used. Knowing how to recognize and work with these differences is what makes home pharmacy practice truly personal.

Taste is one of the most immediate and influential aspects in choosing and using a remedy. Even the best relaxing herbal tea can be ineffective if it tastes so unpleasant as to discourage the drinker. This is where the art of balance comes in: a chamomile infusion can be enhanced with a drizzle of honey or the addition of herbs such as mint, which not only improve the flavor but can also amplify the benefits. The ability to vary the flavor profile of a recipe makes it accessible to a wider range of people, turning a simple remedy into a moment of pleasure.

In addition to taste, personal health conditions play a crucial role in adapting recipes. Not all herbs are suitable for everyone. For example, St. John's Wort, known for its mood benefits, can interact with drugs such as antidepressants, making it an unsafe choice for some. In such cases, an alternative such as passionflower may be more appropriate. Adapting a recipe means knowing not only the effects of the plants, but also the potential risks and contraindications, ensuring that the remedy is safe and effective for the user.

Availability of ingredients also plays a significant role. Not everyone has access to a wide selection of fresh or dried herbs, especially if they live in urban areas or in regions where some plants do not grow easily. However, this does not mean giving up one's ideal remedy. Often, there are substitutions that can maintain the effectiveness of the original recipe. If dandelion is not available, wild chicory can be a viable alternative for its similar purifying properties. Creativity and knowledge of these options allow remedies to be adapted to available resources, ensuring that no need remains unmet.

Adapting also means enhancing what one has on hand, turning common ingredients into valuable solutions. Even a well-stocked kitchen can become a home pharmacy: spices such as ginger, cinnamon, or turmeric, which are readily available, can be the basis of herbal teas and compresses with amazing properties. This approach not only makes remedies more accessible, but also promotes a mindset of self-sufficiency and sustainability.

Ultimately, adapting recipes means putting the person, his or her needs and resources at the center. It is a process of listening and caring, transforming each preparation into a unique remedy that is deeply connected to the user.

HERBAL PROPERTIES: HOW TO COMBINE THEM TO ENHANCE THEIR EFFECT

Herbal properties are at the heart of the home pharmacy. Each plant holds unique potential that can be harnessed in different ways, depending on the combination chosen. Understanding how to combine herbs not only to add up, but also to enhance their effects, is one of the most valuable skills one can develop in this area.

Each herb has one or more main properties. Some are relaxing, some are anti-inflammatory, and some are stimulating or purifying. When you combine several herbs with complementary properties, you can create a synergy that amplifies the desired result. This phenomenon, called the synergistic effect, is the basis for preparing herbal teas, tinctures, and ointments that are more effective than using a single plant.

For example, consider a sleep remedy. Chamomile is widely known for its calming properties, but its effect can be enhanced by adding lemon balm, which acts similarly by reducing anxiety and relaxing the nervous system. Then, if even deeper action is desired, valerian, which has a direct impact on sleep induction, can be included. This combination takes advantage of the relaxing qualities of each plant, creating a more complete and balanced effect.

Similarly, herbs can be combined to address multiple needs in a single remedy. A herbal tea for digestion, for example, may include ginger to stimulate digestion, fennel to reduce bloating, and peppermint to calm any intestinal spasms. Each plant acts on a specific aspect of the problem, but together they work to provide total and rapid relief.

The art of combining herbs also requires knowing their active ingredients. Some plants contain tannins, which can have an astringent and anti-inflammatory effect, while others are rich in mucilage, which is useful for soothing and protecting irritated tissues. By combining these two categories, an effective remedy for problems such as sore throat can be created by combining an astringent plant such as sage with one rich in mucilage, such as mallow. The combined action not only reduces inflammation but also protects the irritated throat, promoting faster healing.

It should not be forgotten that some combinations can improve the absorption of active ingredients. Turmeric, for example, is very effective as a natural anti-inflammatory, but its active ingredient, curcumin, is difficult to absorb on its own. By adding black pepper, which contains piperine, the absorption of curcumin increases significantly, making the remedy much more effective.

However, it is important to remember that not all herbs can be combined without risk. Some plants have similar properties that, when used together in excessive amounts, can cause undesirable effects. Therefore, it is essential to know well the plants you are using, start with low doses and observe how the body reacts. This approach allows you to make the most of the power of herbs, building customized remedies that are both safe and effective.

Combining herbs to enhance their effects is not just a technique, but an art that requires practice, sensitivity, and a deep connection with nature. It is through this process that herbal remedies are transformed from simple preparations into powerful tools for holistic wellness.

Here are some suggestions for combining herbs to enhance their effect, organized according to the main benefits you want to achieve. Each combination takes advantage of the unique properties of individual plants, creating synergies that enhance the effectiveness of the remedy.

1. FOR RELAXATION AND SLEEP
Chamomile + Lemon Balm + Valerian
These herbs work together to calm the mind, relax the nervous system and promote deep sleep. Chamomile and lemon balm reduce anxiety, while valerian acts directly as a natural sedative.
Suggested use: evening herbal teas or tinctures.

Lavender + Passionflower + Linden.
Lavender calms nerves and relieves tension headaches, passionflower reduces irritability, and linden relaxes muscles and promotes rest.
Suggested use: relaxing infusion or massage oil.

2. TO IMPROVE DIGESTION.
Ginger + Fennel + Peppermint.
The perfect trio to support digestion. Ginger stimulates gastric juices, fennel reduces bloating, and mint relaxes stomach muscles, preventing cramping.
Suggested use: post-meal herbal teas or concentrated extracts.

Anise + Coriander + Roman Chamomile.
These herbs work synergistically to combat nausea, improve nutrient absorption, and reduce intestinal inflammation.
Suggested use: digestive infusion or as an addition to dishes.

3. TO STRENGTHEN THE IMMUNE SYSTEM
Echinacea + Rosehip + Ginger.
Echinacea stimulates white blood cell production, rosehip is rich in vitamin C, and ginger adds a powerful anti-inflammatory effect.
Suggested use: tinctures, herbal teas or natural syrups.

Thyme + Sage + Lemon
Thyme is a powerful antibacterial, sage is anti-inflammatory, and lemon provides vitamin C to support natural defenses.
Suggested use: gargle for sore throat or warm herbal tea.

4. FOR ENERGY AND CONCENTRATION
Rosemary + Ginseng + Spearmint.
Rosemary stimulates cerebral circulation, ginseng increases resistance to fatigue, and spearmint provides a freshness that awakens the mind.
Suggested use: morning infusions or essential oils for aromatherapy.

Yerba Mate + Eleutherococcus + Lemon.
This combination offers lasting energy without jitters: yerba mate is a source of natural caffeine, eleutherococcus improves stress resistance, and lemon refreshes.

Suggested use: tea or energy tinctures.

5. TO RELIEVE PAIN AND REDUCE INFLAMMATION.

Devil's claw + turmeric + ginger.

Devil's claw relieves joint pain, turmeric fights chronic inflammation, and ginger improves circulation, enhancing the anti-inflammatory effect.

Suggested use: decoctions or ointments.

White Willow + Arnica + Lavender

White willow, due to its salicin content, is a natural analgesic, arnica relieves muscle pain, and lavender relaxes tense muscles.

Suggested use: warm creams or compresses.

6. FOR RESPIRATORY HEALTH

Eucalyptus + Peppermint + Thyme.

This combination helps clear the respiratory tract: eucalyptus decongests, peppermint soothes, and thyme fights infection.

Suggested use: inhalations or balms.

Licorice + Mallow + Althea

Licorice reduces throat irritation, mallow protects with its mucilage, and marshmallow soothes a dry cough.
Suggested use: syrups or herbal teas.

7. FOR GENERAL WELL-BEING AND DETOXIFICATION

Dandelion + Burdock + Nettle

These herbs work synergistically to cleanse the liver, kidneys, and blood, supporting the natural detoxification process.
Suggested use: draining infusions or concentrated extracts.

Calendula + Yarrow + Chamomile

Calendula promotes cell regeneration, yarrow stimulates lymphatic circulation, and chamomile calms internal inflammation.

Suggested use: herbal teas or regenerating creams.

8. TO IMPROVE SKIN HEALTH

Calendula + Burdock + Viola Tricolor

Calendula promotes healing and calms irritation, burdock purifies the blood by reducing impurities on the skin, and viola tricolor is effective against acne and dermatitis due to its anti-inflammatory properties.

Suggested use: purifying herbal teas, creams or compresses.

Rosehip + Aloe Vera + Roman Chamomile

Rosehip is rich in antioxidants to repair skin, aloe vera moisturizes and soothes, and Roman chamomile reduces redness and inflammation.

Suggested use: face masks, moisturizing lotions or skin oils.

9. TO REGULATE THE MENSTRUAL CYCLE AND RELIEVE PAIN

Yarrow + Sage + Verbena

Yarrow regulates menstrual flow, sage balances hormones, and verbena reduces cramps and stress associated with the cycle. This combination helps both regularize and soothe discomfort.

Suggested use: herbal teas or tinctures.

Fennel + Cinnamon + Ginger.

Fennel relieves bloating and aids digestion, cinnamon stimulates circulation, and ginger reduces menstrual cramps due to its anti-inflammatory properties.

Suggested use: hot decoctions or spicy herbal teas.

10. TO SUPPORT MOOD AND REDUCE STRESS

Hypericum + Hawthorn + Passionflower

Hypericum is known for its antidepressant properties, hawthorn calms the heart, and passionflower relieves anxiety and promotes deep relaxation. Together, they offer both emotional and physical support.

Suggested use: relaxing herbal teas or tinctures.

Lavender + Lemon Balm + Rosemary

Lavender relaxes the mind, lemon balm relieves emotional tension, and rosemary stimulates concentration, creating a balance of relaxation and vitality.

Suggested use: afternoon teas or essential oils for diffusers.

INTERACTIONS: HOW TO AVOID COMBINATIONS THAT CANCEL EFFECTS OR MAY BE HARMFUL

When creating customized herbal remedies, it is critical to consider the possible interactions between the herbs used. Not all combinations are beneficial, and some may even nullify desired effects or cause unwanted reactions. Knowing these dynamics is essential to ensure that remedies are safe and effective.

Herbs contain active ingredients that, when combined incorrectly, can compete with each other or have opposite effects. For example, St. John's Wort, known for its antidepressant properties, is a potent enzyme inducer. This means it can speed up the metabolism of some drugs or other plants, reducing their effectiveness. A remedy containing St. John's Wort and valerian, for example, may be less effective, as St. John's Wort may alter the bioavailability of valerian.

Another common example involves herbs that affect the nervous system. Mixing plants with sedative properties, such as valerian, passion flower, and hops, can cause excessive relaxation, leading to drowsiness or reduced alertness, especially if the remedy is taken in high doses or in combination with alcohol or sedative drugs. This effect can be dangerous for those driving or operating machinery.

Herbs with diuretic properties also require attention. Plants such as dandelion or nettle, when used together in high amounts, can lead to excessive electrolyte loss, causing imbalances in the body. It is important to balance these effects by adding herbs that replenish minerals, such as burdock or licorice.

In addition to undesirable effects, there are herbs that simply do not work well together. For example, combining plants with astringent properties, such as sage or yarrow, with mucilage-rich herbs, such as mallow or marshmallow, can reduce the effectiveness of both. Astringent properties tend to "dry out" tissues, while mucilages coat and moisturize them. Using them together can negate the benefits of both categories.

Another risk is the use of herbs that amplify certain effects. For example, ginseng and the natural caffeine in yerba mate or green tea can overstimulate the nervous system, leading to nervousness, anxiety, or palpitations if used together without care. Similarly, plants such as ginkgo biloba, which improve circulation, could interact with other anticoagulant herbs, such as garlic or ginger, increasing the risk of bleeding.

To avoid problematic combinations, it is important to follow a few key rules. First, study the individual properties of the herbs and understand their mechanism of action. Using reliable sources or consulting herbal experts can help identify potential interactions. Second, always start with small amounts and carefully observe the body's reactions, avoiding combining many herbs in one preparation, especially if you are inexperienced.

Jotting down one's preparations can also be very helpful. Keeping a recipe diary, with details of ingredients used, doses, and effects experienced, allows you to monitor the effectiveness of combinations and identify any problems. Finally, it is always advisable to avoid combining herbs with medications without first consulting a qualified physician or herbalist.

With a careful and informed approach, it is possible to avoid harmful interactions and create herbal remedies that are safe, effective, and harmonious.

Here are 10 examples of herbal combinations that are best avoided, accompanied by the reasons why these associations are problematic:

1. HYPERICUM + VALERIAN
Rationale: St. John's Wort can speed up the metabolism of valerian, reducing its effectiveness. Also, both act on the nervous system and may cause excessive sedative effect if taken together.

2. GINKGO BILOBA + GINGER + GARLIC
Rationale: All of these herbs have anticoagulant properties. Taking them together may increase the risk of bleeding, especially for those who take anticoagulant drugs or have clotting problems.

3. SAGE + MALLOW
Rationale: Sage has astringent properties, while mallow is rich in mucilage that moisturizes and coats tissues. Using them together can negate the benefits of both, as their actions are opposite.

4. GINSENG + YERBA MATE + GREEN TEA.
Rationale: These herbs stimulate the nervous system and, when combined, can lead to overstimulation, causing anxiety, nervousness, palpitations or insomnia.

5. DANDELION + NETTLE
Rationale: Both are diuretics. Taking them together can cause excessive loss of fluids and electrolytes, leading to imbalances that could be harmful to the body.

6. LICORICE + HYPERICUM
Rationale: Licorice may increase blood pressure, while St. John's Wort may interfere with antihypertensive medications. The combination could cause pressure imbalances or interfere with blood pressure control.

7. LAVENDER + HOPS + PASSIONFLOWER
Rationale: All of these herbs have sedative effects. Taking them together in large amounts can lead to excessive drowsiness, difficulty concentrating and, in some cases, dizziness.

8. GINKGO BILOBA + GINSENG
Rationale: Ginkgo biloba stimulates cerebral circulation, while ginseng is energizing. The combination can cause mental overexcitement, nervousness or, in extreme cases, headaches.

9. CHAMOMILE + ECHINACEA
Rationale: Both can cause allergic reactions in sensitive people, especially those allergic to plants in the Asteraceae family. Taking them together increases the risk of adverse reactions.

10. TURMERIC + BLACK PEPPER (IN EXCESSIVE AMOUNTS).
Rationale: Although black pepper enhances the absorption of curcumin found in turmeric, an excessive amount may cause gastric irritation or gastrointestinal problems, especially in sensitive people.

SUBSTITUTIONS: COMMON ALTERNATIVES WHEN AN INGREDIENT IS NOT AVAILABLE

Substitutions are an essential part of home pharmacy practice. It is not always possible to have access to all the herbs needed for a prescription, but this should not become an obstacle. There are many viable substitutions that make it possible to maintain the effectiveness of a remedy by adapting it to available resources or personal needs. Knowing these substitutions means being able to work more flexibly and creatively, without compromising results.

When an ingredient is not available, the first step is to consider its purpose in the recipe. For example, if an herb is used for its calming properties, it is important to choose a substitute that has similar effects. Adapting a remedy means not just substituting an ingredient, but doing so with awareness, maintaining the right balance among the elements in the preparation.

A classic example is chamomile, often used for relaxation and sleep. If it is not available, other herbs such as lemon balm or passion flower can be substituted without problem. Both have similar relaxing properties and offer a mild flavor profile, making them ideal for evening infusions.

Another common case involves turmeric, known for its anti-inflammatory properties. If turmeric is not available, ginger can be a viable alternative. Although the two plants have different active ingredients, they share anti-inflammatory effects and are both readily available. In addition, ginger adds a spicy note that can enrich many recipes.

For remedies that require plants with astringent properties, such as sage or yarrow, you can use horsetail or rose hips as substitutes. Both have similar effects, helping to tone tissues and reduce inflammation, with added unique benefits such as skin support or immune system strengthening.

Substitutions are not limited to herbs. Solvents used in tinctures can also be adapted. For example, if you do not have food alcohol for a tincture, you can use apple cider vinegar or vegetable glycerin. These solvents are less potent in extracting some active ingredients, but they are safe and practical alternatives, especially for those who prefer to avoid alcohol.

The soothing properties of mucilage-rich plants, such as mallow or marshmallow, can be replicated with the use of flaxseed. Preparing an infusion of flaxseed yields a mucilage-rich solution that can be used to soothe internal or external irritation.

Carrier oils can also be substituted easily. If a recipe calls for jojoba oil but it is not available, sweet almond oil or coconut oil are good alternatives. These oils are nourishing and light, and can be used for skin or hair without overly altering the preparation.

The flexibility offered by substitutions also makes herbalism accessible to those who do not have a large supply of ingredients. Experimenting with alternatives not only broadens the possibilities, but also allows new combinations and properties to be discovered, making each remedy unique and personal. With time and experience, this adaptability becomes a valuable tool for anyone who wants to practice home pharmacy with confidence and creativity.

Here are 10 examples of common home pharmacy substitutions that will allow you to adapt recipes even when you do not have the original ingredient on hand:

1. CHAMOMILE → LEMON BALM OR PASSIONFLOWER
When to substitute: For herbal teas or relaxing remedies.
Rationale: Lemon balm and passionflower have similar calming properties and help reduce anxiety and promote sleep.

2. TURMERIC → GINGER
When to substitute: For anti-inflammatory recipes.
Rationale: Ginger shares the anti-inflammatory properties of turmeric and is also a good digestive stimulant.

3. LAVENDER → LIME OR ROMAN CHAMOMILE.

When to substitute: For relaxing infusions or essential oils.
Rationale: Lime and Roman chamomile offer similar calming effects and a mild aroma profile.

4. SAGE → YARROW OR HORSETAIL.

When to substitute: For astringent or tonic properties.
Rationale: Yarrow and horsetail can help tone tissues and reduce inflammation, offering similar benefits.

5. ROSEHIP → HIBISCUS

When to substitute: For herbal teas rich in vitamin C.
Rationale: Hibiscus has a high vitamin C content and a similar tart taste, ideal for supporting the immune system.

6. HYPERICUM → HAWTHORN

When to substitute: For anxiety remedies or mood support.
Rationale: Hawthorn calms the nervous system and promotes a feeling of well-being, while being safer for those taking medications.

7. PEPPERMINT → SPEARMINT OR FENNEL.

When to substitute: For digestive herbal teas.
Rationale: Spearmint and fennel have similar properties in relaxing stomach muscles and improving digestion.

8. JOJOBA OIL → SWEET ALMOND OIL OR COCONUT OIL.

When to substitute: For massage oils or skin conditioners.
Rationale: Both oils are nourishing, light and well tolerated by most skin.

9. ALTHEA → MALLOW OR FLAXSEED.

When to substitute: To soothe internal inflammation or irritation.
Rationale: Mallow and flaxseed release mucilage that protects and moisturizes irritated tissues.

10. ECHINACEA → DANDELION OR BURDOCK.

When to substitute: To support the immune system.
Rationale: Dandelion and burdock have purifying effects on the body and indirectly support the immune system through detoxification.

BASIC RULES FOR CREATING A BALANCED BLEND

Creating a balanced blend is an art that requires care, knowledge of herb properties, and a systematic approach. Each herb in a blend should have a well-defined role, contributing to the overall effectiveness without overwhelming the others. By following some basic rules, it is possible to formulate balanced and potent remedies that are safe, effective, and pleasant to use.

1. DEFINE THE PURPOSE OF THE MIXTURE

Before you begin, it is important to clarify what problem or goal you want to address with the blend. For example, a relaxing herbal tea will have a different focus than a blend to improve digestion or relieve a cold. This helps in choosing the main herbs that will form the basis of the remedy.

2. CHOOSE A "MAIN HERB"

The main herb is the key element of the mixture, the one that determines the desired effect. It should make up about 40-60% of the total mixture. For example, if you are creating an herbal tea for sleep, chamomile or valerian could be the main herbs. Their action will drive the final result.

3. ADD "SUPPORT" HERBS

Supporting herbs reinforce or amplify the effect of the main herb. They must complement and work synergistically with the main ingredient. These herbs make up about 20-30% of the blend. For a relaxing herbal tea, you might add lemon balm or linden to enhance the calming effect.

4. INCLUDE "AROMATIC" OR "SECONDARY" HERBS.

Aromatic herbs enhance the taste, aroma, and overall experience of the blend. Although they do not play a major role in the therapeutic effect, they can make the remedy more pleasant to take. These herbs make up about 10-20% of the mixture. Mint, orange peel, or cinnamon are good examples for adding aroma and flavor.

5. PAY ATTENTION TO THE BALANCE OF FLAVORS AND PROPERTIES

A balanced blend should not only be effective, but also pleasant. Too bitter, too sweet, or too astringent can make it difficult to take the remedy. A good balance of flavors (sweet, spicy, bitter, sour) can enhance the sensory experience. For example, a mixture with bitter herbs such as yarrow could be balanced by adding licorice to sweeten the taste.

6. CONSIDER DOSES AND POTENCY

It is essential to use herbs in the right amounts to avoid unwanted effects. For example, some herbs, such as valerian or ginseng, can be potent even in small doses. A rule of thumb is to start with small doses and gradually increase only if necessary. Noting down any variations will help refine the mixture over time.

7. EVALUATE PREPARATION TIME

Each herb requires a specific infusion or steeping time to extract its active ingredients. It is important to choose herbs with similar preparation times or adjust the preparation to ensure that all plants effectively release their benefits. For example, if some herbs require short infusion and others long, you can add them at different times during preparation.

8. MAINTAIN A RECIPE LOG

A journal or blending log is essential for perfecting your preparations. Jot down the ingredients, proportions, preparation methods, and results obtained. This will help you replicate a successful blend or modify it to improve results.

EXAMPLE OF A BALANCED BLEND FOR RELAXATION:

Main herb: Chamomile (40%)
Supporting herbs: Lemon balm (30%) and Linden (20%)
Aromatic herb: Peppermint (10%)

This relaxing blend is balanced in both taste and effectiveness, with herbs working synergistically to calm the mind and relax the body.

By following these basic rules, each blend will be the result of a thoughtful and harmonious combination, ready to deliver the desired benefits with confidence and taste.

TECHNIQUES FOR SAFE EXPERIMENTATION

Experimenting with herbal remedies is a fascinating part of home pharmacy practice, but it is critical to do so safely. Plants are powerful healing tools, and an informed approach reduces the risk of unwanted effects or dangerous interactions. By following a few key techniques, you can explore new combinations and customizations without compromising your own or others' well-being.

1. START WITH ONE HERB AT A TIME

When experimenting with a new herb, it is advisable to use it alone before adding it to a more complex mixture. This allows you to assess how your body reacts and identify any side effects or sensitivities. For example, before incorporating valerian into a sleep herbal tea, try using it alone to test its relaxing effect and make sure it does not cause excessive drowsiness or dizziness.

2. USE SMALL AMOUNTS

When trying a new combination or preparation that has never been tested, start with small doses. This approach minimizes risk and allows you to evaluate the effectiveness of the remedy. For an herbal tea, for example, use a teaspoon of dried herb instead of a tablespoon, observing the effects before gradually increasing the dose.

3. DOCUMENT EACH ATTEMPT

Keeping a journal of your experiments is an indispensable tool. Record the herbs used, quantities, methods of preparation, and effects found. If a combination proves particularly effective or you notice unwanted reactions, this information will help you replicate or modify the mixture with awareness.

4. KNOW THE PROPERTIES OF HERBS

Before using a plant, study its properties, active ingredients and possible contraindications. Some herbs may interact with medications or specific health conditions. For example, St. John's Wort may reduce the effectiveness of some antidepressant or contraceptive medications. Knowing this information allows you to avoid mistakes and unsafe experimentation.

5. COMBINE A FEW HERBS AT A TIME

When creating a blend, limit the number of herbs used, especially if you are experimenting with new combinations. A mixture with 2-3 herbs is easier to manage than one with 5-6, and allows you to more easily identify which ingredient is working or causing side effects.

6. TRY HERBS IN DIFFERENT PREPARATION METHODS

Herbs can act in different ways depending on the method of preparation. A plant used in infusion may have milder effects than the same plant in tincture or decoction. Experimenting with different methods helps you discover the most effective mode for a given remedy.

7. RESPECT TRIAL TIMES

Give your body time to get used to a new remedy before judging its effectiveness. Many herbs, such as echinacea or turmeric, require regular use for a few weeks before they show their full benefits. However, if you notice immediate side effects, discontinue use immediately and take note of reactions.

8. WATCH OUT FOR ALLERGIC REACTIONS

Even the most common herbs can cause allergic reactions in some people. If you are trying a new plant, start with a minimal amount and watch for any signs of reaction, such as itching, swelling or difficulty breathing. If allergy symptoms appear, stop use immediately and, if necessary, consult a doctor.

9. AVOID COMBINATIONS WITH EXCESSIVE SIMILAR EFFECTS

When experimenting with blends, be careful not to combine herbs that have similar, overly intense effects. For example, avoid mixing too many sedative herbs, such as valerian, hops, and passion flower, as they may cause excessive drowsiness or dizziness. Always balance the effects of herbs to achieve a harmonious remedy.

10. CONSULT RELIABLE RESOURCES

When exploring new herbs or techniques, rely on credible sources of information such as herbal books, scientific studies or courses with experts. If you have doubts, consulting a qualified herbalist or doctor is always a good idea, especially for remedies intended for children, the elderly, or people with special health conditions.

By following these techniques, experimenting becomes a safe and rewarding process. The gradual, mindful approach not only reduces risks, but also allows you to hone your skills, developing personalized remedies that meet your specific needs.

CUSTOMIZING RECIPES FOR CHILDREN OR SENSITIVE PEOPLE

Customizing recipes for children or sensitive people requires a delicate and targeted approach. These groups have specific needs and a greater vulnerability to the effects of certain herbal remedies, which is why it is essential to adapt dosages, herbs, and methods of preparation. With proper care, you can create safe and effective recipes that respect their particular sensitivities.

1. ADAPT DOSAGES
The first rule when preparing remedies for children or sensitive people is to reduce the dosage from the standard dosage for an adult. For children, a good rule of thumb is to use a proportionate dosage based on weight. For example, a child who weighs one-third of an adult should receive about one-third of the dosage. For sensitive people, such as the elderly or those with a petite build, it is always best to start with a low dose and increase gradually, monitoring the effects.

2. CHOOSE HERBS THAT ARE GENTLE AND SAFE
Not all herbs are suitable for children or people with particular sensitivities. Prefer plants with a safe and well-documented profile. For example:

- **Chamomile**: Perfect for calming nerves, relieving stomach upset and promoting sleep.
- **Lemon Balm**: Relaxing and gentle, ideal for agitated children or anxious people.
- **Linden**: Useful for reducing mild fever or calming respiratory ailments.
- **Calendula**: Safe for topical application, soothes skin irritations and minor cuts.

Instead, avoid powerful or stimulating herbs such as St. John's Wort, ephedra or ginseng, which may be too strong or have unexpected side effects.

3. USE LESS CONCENTRATED METHODS OF PREPARATION
For children or sensitive people, it is advisable to prepare less concentrated remedies. For example, an herbal tea for an adult might require one tablespoon of herbs per cup, but for a child half a teaspoon is sufficient. For tinctures, however, opt for vegetable glycerin instead of alcohol, which is gentler and tastes better.

4. CHOOSE PALATABLE METHODS OF ADMINISTRATION
Taste is important, especially for children. To make remedies more palatable:

Add honey (for children over 12 months) or maple syrup to herbal teas.
Make sweetened herbal syrups, ideal for relieving coughs or sore throats.
Use diluted essential oils for massage or diffusers, rather than herbal teas or tinctures, to avoid direct ingestion.
For sensitive people, you can opt for controlled-release capsules or aromatic herbal teas, which offer a pleasant and less invasive experience.

5. ADAPT RECIPES FOR COMMON AILMENTS
Here are some recipes adapted for children and sensitive people:

Calming Sleep Infusion:
Chamomile (1 part), Lemon Balm (1 part), Lavender (half teaspoon per cup).
Method: let steep for 5-7 minutes. Sweeten lightly with honey.
Dosage: half cup for children, one cup for sensitive adults.

Soothing skin bath:
Dried Calendula (2 tablespoons), Mallow (1 tablespoon).
Method: prepare a decoction and add it to bath water.
Use: good for soothing dermatitis or rashes.

THE ART OF HOME APOTHECARY

Relaxing massage oil:
Sweet almond oil (50 ml), 2 drops lavender essential oil.
Method: mix ingredients and apply with gentle massage.
Use: ideal for soothing children before bedtime or relaxing adults with sensitive skin.

6. MONITOR AND ADAPT REACTIONS

When creating remedies for children or sensitive people, carefully monitor their reactions. Signs of discomfort, such as skin redness or gastrointestinal upset, are indicative that a remedy may not be suitable. It is important to note this information and adjust future preparations accordingly.

7. AVOID PROBLEMATIC CATEGORIES OF HERBS.

Some herbs are generally not recommended for children and sensitive people. Avoid stimulant plants (such as guarana or green coffee), powerful purgatives (such as internal aloe vera) or those with a lesser known safety profile. Always favor the most studied and safest options.

With these steps, you can create customized herbal remedies that respect the needs of children and sensitive people, ensuring that they have a positive and safe experience with home pharmacy.

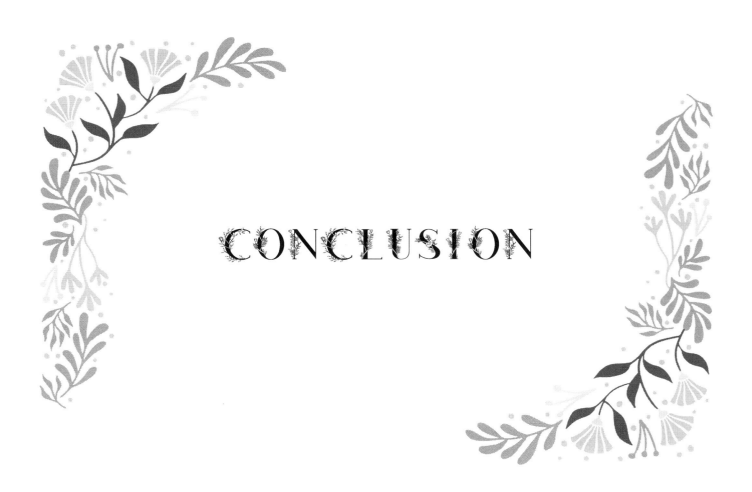

CONCLUSION

CHAPTER 13:
THE FUTURE OF THE HOME APOTHECARY

FINAL ENCOURAGEMENT - INTEGRATING THE HOME APOTHECARY INTO DAILY LIFE

Creating and maintaining a home pharmacy is a journey that goes far beyond simply growing and preparing natural remedies. It is a journey that weaves together self-care, sustainability and a deep connection with nature. Integrating this practice into your daily life does not mean disrupting habits, but rather enriching them, turning every gesture into an opportunity to take care of your body and mind with simple and natural tools.

Home pharmacy can become a personal or family ritual, a time for reflection and mindful attention. Preparing a relaxing herbal tea in the evening, massaging your skin with a homemade infused oil, or simply breathing in the aroma of dried herbs can become daily gestures that anchor your routine in a sense of calm and well-being. Each time you use a remedy you have created with your own hands, you are choosing to move closer to a more natural lifestyle, celebrating self-sufficiency and respect for what nature has to offer.

Integrating home pharmacy into everyday life begins with small steps. You do not need to create a vast repertoire of remedies right away or cultivate a complete botanical garden. You can start with a few commonly used herbs and a few simple preparations, such as a tincture of chamomile for relaxation or a calendula salve for irritated skin. Over time, this practice will expand naturally, following your needs and curiosity.

Another important aspect is to involve the people around you. Sharing an herbal tea with a friend, giving a homemade ointment as a gift, or explaining the benefits of herbs can inspire others to take this path. Home pharmacy is not only an act of personal care, but also a way to build community and pass on valuable knowledge. Every recipe, every plant grown, every remedy created becomes part of a legacy that you can share with future generations.

Finally, integrating home pharmacy into your life means embracing a mindset of continuous learning. Each season, each harvest, and each new preparation presents an opportunity to discover something new. Even when some experiments do not go as planned, the process itself is an enriching experience. Nature is a generous ally, always ready to teach us, as long as we stop to listen.

The future of home pharmacy is bright, especially at a time when the desire for sustainability and natural health is on the rise. With patience, dedication and a little creativity, you can make home pharmacy not only a resource for your health, but also a way to live more in tune with the world around you.

SHARING KNOWLEDGE - HOW TO PASS DOWN TRADITIONS AND NATURAL PRACTICES

Home pharmacy is not only an individual practice, but also an opportunity to make connections and pass on valuable knowledge. Traditions related to the use of medicinal herbs have survived for centuries through sharing, from the wise herbalists of the past to the families who passed down recipes and secrets from one generation to the next. Today, in an age dominated by technology, sharing these practices can not only preserve them but also inspire a return to nature and a more conscious lifestyle.

Sharing your knowledge can take many forms, all equally meaningful. It can start with small gestures, such as talking about the beneficial properties of herbs with friends and family. Making herbal tea together, showing how to dry plants or explaining how to make an ointment can be moments of connection that strengthen personal bonds. These simple acts convey the importance of self-care and respect for nature in a practical and direct way.

Another way to share knowledge is to involve children. Growing herbs together with them, teaching the names of plants and telling stories about their properties not only stimulates their curiosity but also brings them closer to nature. Children are naturally fascinated by plants and the processes of transformation, such as seeing a fresh plant become a tincture or herbal tea. This kind of hands-on learning leaves a lasting impression and can inspire a lifelong love of botany and natural health.

If you want to expand sharing further, consider organizing small workshops or informal gatherings for your community. You could show how to make a healing salve, create a vertical garden, or explain the safe use of tinctures. Even if you are not a recognized expert, your passion and commitment can make a difference. These meetings are opportunities to exchange ideas, experiences and knowledge, creating a network of people who share the same interest in home pharmacy.

Another modern form of transmission is digital sharing. Blogs, social media, and video tutorials provide a platform to reach a wider audience. Documenting your experiences, sharing recipes, and recounting the successes and challenges of your journey can inspire others around the world. Transparency and authenticity are keys to engaging those who are new to the practice and making it accessible even to those who have never considered starting a home pharmacy.

Finally, don't forget to leave a tangible record of your journey. This can be a journal in which you jot down recipes, observations about plants, and methods you have found most effective. This journal can be shared with your loved ones, becoming a living legacy that will continue to inspire future generations. It can become a personal guide, enriched by your experience, encapsulating your knowledge and discoveries.

Sharing knowledge is not just about teaching others; it is also about building an ongoing learning community, where ideas and inspiration flow in both directions. Every time you pass on a practice or knowledge, you are helping to keep an ancient tradition alive and strengthen the bond between humans and nature. Home pharmacy is not just a personal treasure: it is a gift that can grow and enrich anyone who is willing to receive it.

THE ART OF HOME APOTHECARY

Made in United States
Orlando, FL
17 May 2025

61369845R00103